EARTH TREASURES

A FOCUSED JOURNEY INTO THE FOUNDATION OF AROMATHERAPY

Volume Two

Editor:
James Barker [creativeunit@gmail.com]
Anne Karklins [anne@hasmarkpublishing.com]

Cover Design:
James Barker [creativeunit@gmail.com]

Interior Layout:
James Barker [creativeunit@gmail.com]

ISBN 13: 979-8-9911716-4-9

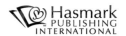

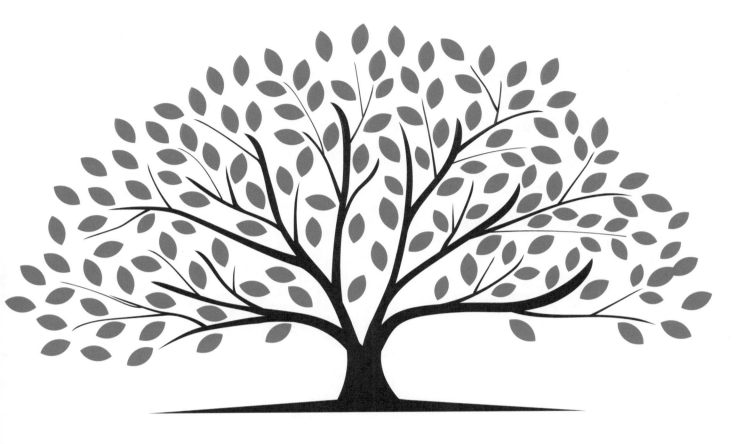

Volume Two

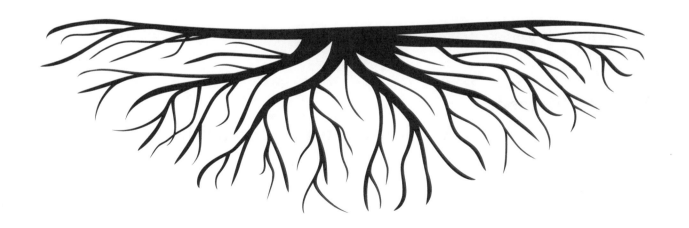

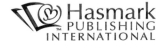

Hasmark
PUBLISHING
INTERNATIONAL

CONTENTS

Chapter Fifteen:

FORWARD by Dr. Patrick Porter, Ph.D.

I remember meeting Dr. Zepf many years ago in Hawaii and questioning her about the benefits of essential oils. As she explained the science behind essential oils and her processes to preserve and create the best quality products, I knew that this was someone that I could learn from and develop an awareness of essential oils with that I wouldn't have gotten from anyone else.

She helped to guide us through how to test through our NeuralChek technology, how essential oils actually affect brain function, and how to use them in clinical settings. As I shared this information with the over 3000 doctors in our BrainTap community, they all became excited about Dr. Zepf's knowledge and information.

I'm so pleased that she's now put all of her wisdom into this book to share with more of the world. I'll be sharing the title with everyone I know so they can benefit from what she's sharing as well. I believe that Dr. Zepf is on the cutting edge in training people not only useful information regarding essential oils, but the value of properly sourcing the materials through proper application and explaining it to clients. She has a full soup to nuts experience where someone can come in without knowing much at all about essential oils and they can come out the other end being proficient and can then give the same quality of care that Dr. Zepf gives her own clients.

It's a rare person that can take their knowledge which they've worked years to compile in personal practice and then share that with the world so they too can be empowered not to have to go through the learning curve of ten, 20 or even 30 years to master the topic of essential oils. So congratulations, Dr. Zefp for doing that.

And to you, the reader, congratulations for picking this book up and wanting to learn and develop a primal sense of smell and in taking this ancient tradition and transforming it into a modern technology-- a technique that can be used by any practitioner, whether it be for wellbeing or for serenity. Whatever the need, there is an essential oil that can benefit and Dr. Zepf can train you to understand the benefits of using this olfactory feature—which most therapies leave out of the equation.

As a neuroscientist, I understand the more we can involve the different senses in the transformation and change of our clients. the better off we're all going to be at the end of the day. The goal is to help clients be successful, to build better practices and eventually a better world. So I invite you to enjoy what you're about to read. Years of blood, sweat and tears went in to the creation of these pages and believe me when I say this is only scratching the surface of what Dr. Zepf can teach you.

Once you're done she'll give you direction on where to go from here to continue to accelerate your learning and the benefits of using essential oils.

Neurologically yours,

♠ **Dr. Patrick Porter, PhD**
Inventor and Founder of BrainTap Technology

With over 35 years of entrepreneurial experience in the health, wellness, and personal development industry, Dr. Patrick K. Porter has established himself as a leading figure in brainwave entrainment technology and neuroscience research.

Dr. Porter's distinguished career is marked by his innovative approach to brainwave entrainment and his dedication to improving mental and physical health through groundbreaking technology and research collaborations, such as the one with AIIMS Bhopal, which earned international recognition.

BLENDING PRINCIPLES

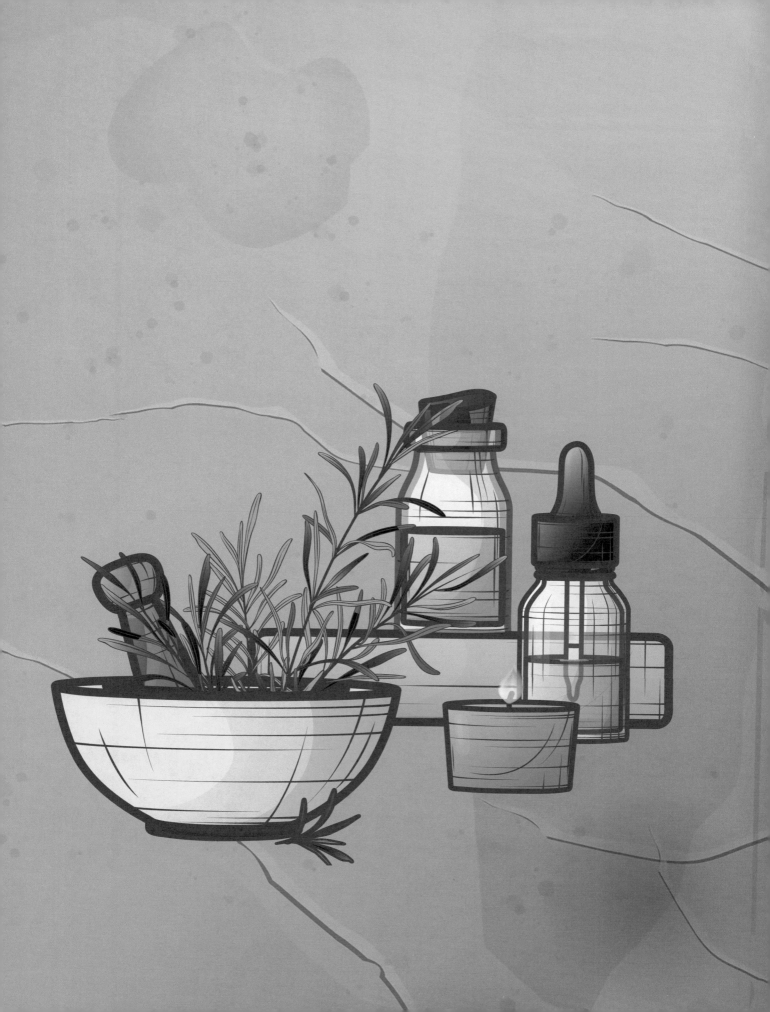

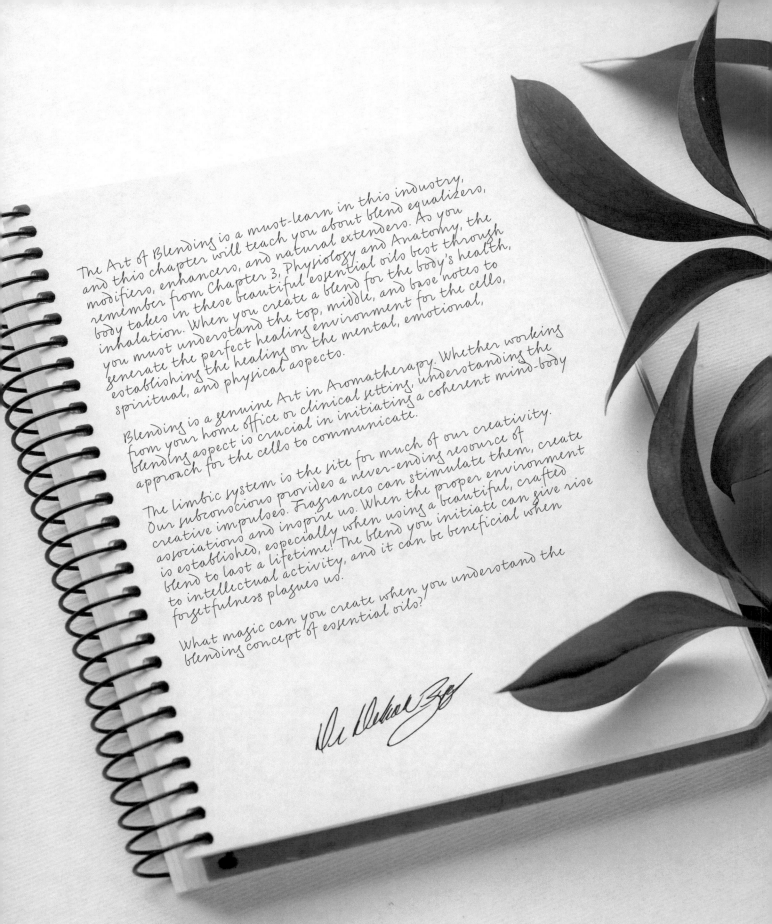

The Art of Blending is a must-learn in this industry, and this chapter will teach you about blend equalizers, modifiers, enhancers, and natural extenders. As you remember from Chapter 3, Physiology and Anatomy, the body takes in these beautiful essential oils best through inhalation. When you create a blend for the body's health, you must understand the top, middle, and base notes to generate the perfect healing environment for the cells, establishing the healing on the mental, emotional, spiritual, and physical aspects.

Blending is a genuine Art in Aromatherapy. Whether working from your home office or clinical setting, understanding the blending aspect is crucial in initiating a coherent mind-body approach for the cells to communicate.

The limbic system is the site for much of our creativity. Our subconscious provides a never-ending resource of creative impulses. Fragrances can stimulate them, create associations and inspire us. When the proper environment is established, especially when using a beautiful, crafted blend to last a lifetime! The blend you initiate can give rise to intellectual activity, and it can be beneficial when forgetfulness plagues us.

What magic can you create when you understand the blending concept of essential oils?

Dr. Deborah Bks

CHAPTER TWELVE:
BLENDING PRINCIPLES

Blending requires the full knowledge of essential oils, from background and history to chemical composition to human physiology and mental wellness. Only through knowledge, education, practical experience, and building intuition can a practitioner discern the most effective blends and uses for essential oils. Intuition and experience are developed over time, through trial and error, and are intrinsic skills to create a purposeful, effective blend.

Because differences in body systems, as well as the user's personal preference, can influence each blend's effectiveness, learning to develop supportive blends is as much an art as it is a science. The blend that supports health and wellness in one individual who embraces the scent and healing vibrations may be a total failure to someone else who rejects the blend because of smell or simple dislike. If the combination does not create synergy with the patient, the healing will not occur or will be minimal.

To create an effective, synergistic blend, each practitioner must understand and address the symptoms that must be treated to bring the body back to balance and the underlying causes. Often, the symptoms mask the root cause of imbalances, and careful research through questions and testing may be needed to identify and treat the underlying cause. Until the root cause is identified, new and seemingly unrelated symptoms may continue to appear.

> "When creating a blend, first look at the purpose of the mixture. A blend to fight infection will be very different from one to soothe emotional wounds or to relieve stress. An infection-fighting blend will be built like a small commando of very efficient, no-nonsense soldiers. You want to get the job done as quickly and cleanly as possible. Your main concern is that the purpose is clear and that all oils used work very disciplined towards the same goal.
> The fragrance is secondary.
>
> For emotional problems on the other hand, fragrance is of utmost importance, and you will need to carefully and skillfully build your blend to produce a pleasant one."

Marcel Levabre [1]

Blending allows you to express your creative energies and skills. Thoughtfulness and creativity play an essential role in creating a powerful, dynamic, and synergistic blend that will enhance the effectiveness of the treatment.

For example, arthritic pain is a frequent complaint from patients. However, the pain and arthritis conditions are often not the root cause. Through research, a patient's condition may be identified as rheumatoid arthritis. On a fundamental level, rheumatoid arthritis is an inflammatory response. The following oils provide support for inflammation:

- German Chamomile
- Helichrysum

In researching the symptoms of arthritis, an immediate note should be that all arthritic conditions are accompanied by joint pain. To provide pain relief and support, an essential oil that has analgesic properties to blend might include:

- Ginger
- Cajeput
- Clove

The holistic approach seeks to balance the overall body chemistry, which will alleviate many of the patient's complaints. In addition to balancing chemistry, toxins must be removed from the body to support healing. Detoxification is based on essential oils that support the removal of toxins from the cells of the body, including:

- Juniper Berry
- Carrot Seed
- Sweet Fennel
- Lemon

The immune system can be supported by utilizing monoterpenes in the blend. The blend might be similar to this:

Essential Oil	Principle Constituent	Action	Percentage
thyme (red)	phenol	antimicrobial	20%
hyssop	ketone	mucolytic	20%
sandalwood	sesquiterpenes	anti-inflammatory	10%
eucalyptus radiata	oxide	expectorant	30%
sweet orange	monoterpenes	immunostimulant	20%

(Battaglia)[2]

Many different components are necessary to create a blend that supports the entire body's healing. The foundation of blending is to understand each essential oil's chemistry and psychology fully, but the art of blending goes so much further.

Marcel Lavabre recommends creating blends that treat only a few symptoms and conditions rather than building a blend to treat everything at once. [1] Too many essential oils in a single application will confuse the body systems and cause possible cell contradictions, which prevents healing. The essential oils must work synergistically together. If more conditions need to be addressed, then creating one blend for use at night and one for the morning will allow the separation of oils and provide effective support.

Knowledge of the chemical constituents will be beneficial in creating a blend that creates synergy through each of the component oils. As an example, rosemary essential oil can be very simple or complex, based on which substance is used in the blend.

This chapter explains how to blend an oil and what it means to incorporate a top note, middle note, and base note. It also explains the difference between a single note and a blend of notes. The text will describe the steps to create our very own healing blend, using safety precautions, blending expertise, and making it fit-for-purpose (knowing the conditions to treat and providing an effective essential oil blend for support).

Blending Safety Reminders

Chapter 6 provides detailed safety guidelines, and it is important to review the safety rules of all essential oils before blending. The following safety considerations cover general guidelines (in addition to those specific to the properties of the oils) when blending and when working daily with essential oils:

- Avoid direct contact with pure oils. Always wear gloves.
- Ensure adequate ventilation. Remember, essential oils are volatile, and volatile organic compounds may be inhaled. Direct inhalation can lead to overdosing with dizziness, weakness, and/or nausea symptoms.
- Take frequent breaks. Walk outside into the open air if spending more than 20 minutes blending.
- Avoid touching face/skin, especially around eyes, lips, etc.

Other general cautions when blending and prescribing include:

- Always perform an initial check and second review of the client's medical history
- Do not prescribe the application of essential oils in the armpit area, especially after shaving
- Avoid citrus peel, calamus, or sassafras for clients presenting symptoms or history of melanoma, pre-melanoma patches, large moles, extensive dark freckles, skin cancer, or loss of cognitive ability (related to aging).

Avoid any essential oil before or after strenuous exercise because perspiration may cause increased absorption.

Essential oils are a hundred times stronger than the plant itself. As an example, one drop of peppermint essential oil is equal to approximately 20 cups of tea. The molecular structure has to be broken down for the body to be able to use it correctly and safely.

Robert Tisserand and Tony Balacs have written a comprehensive, detailed book called *"Essential Oil Safety – A Guide for Healthcare Professionals."* This publication provides detailed descriptions of lethal dosages and oral toxicities, safety advice, regulatory guidelines, and organ-specific and systemic effects for many common oils and their chemical constituents. While Chapter 6 provides many safety guidelines, this book is an essential reference for the aromatherapy practitioner's everyday use.

Dilutions

The directions for dilutions are provided in Chapter 6 – Safety. However, these safety notes should always be kept in mind:

- ♠ For a 10ml bottle, creating a 10% dilution means including 1 ml – or 30 drops – in the bottle of your blend and 9 ml – or 270 drops – in the bottle of carrier oil, which creates a 10% dilution.
- ♠ A 5% dilution would be 15 drops in 285 drops or 91/2 ml.
- ♠ A 1% dilution is normally used for children. To create the right dilution, add from 1 drop to 3 drops in 10 ml of oil. Children and the elderly are more sensitive and should receive no more than this 1% dilution for safety reasons.
- ♠ Animals/pets should also be prescribed a 1% dilution.

A Single Note vs. a Blend

The definition of a single note is an oil that is pure with no other essential oils added to it. For example, lavender or rosemary would be considered a single note. Single notes can provide excellent relief for headaches or pain, depending on the situation and the oil prescribed. As described in Chapter 11, a single note may contain over 100 chemical constituents to support the body with healing – allowing the body systems to utilize whatever needed components from those 100 properties. Sometimes, the body will become accustomed to the constituents, or the liver will begin to filter specific components from the blood, and the oil may not provide the same levels of support. Similar mechanisms can occur with medications prescribed for high blood pressure, cholesterol, thyroid, or mental health conditions that suddenly cease effective treatment of symptoms.

When essential oils are blended, the combination then provides as many as 300, 500, and up to 700 different molecular structures to be used at the right time, in its proper sequence, in its right place, and in the right amount. Thus, blends offer greater possibilities and often more support than a single oil. Some specific criteria may respond better to a single note, such as a patient that presents with many allergies. However, a blend allows the practitioner to offer more avenues of support to multiple conditions at the same time.

Picking the Right Oils to Blend

Some oils do not mix well together due to their specific gravity or scent. As an example, benzoin is highly viscous (thick) and will "float" on the top of a blend. When mixed with another oil, it must be emulsified and will still separate over time. It is a very, very heavy oil, and Vetiver has comparable properties.

Also, when creating a blend, contraindications to medicines and specific health conditions are an important consideration to support your clients' wellness. Both patient history and current health conditions must be considered, and any changes should be gathered/reviewed with every appointment (such as an intake form to identify any changes in symptoms, medications, or supplements). This is why blends are usually very personal and best tailored to each patient's specific needs.

Top, Middle, and Base Notes

Four foundational books for an aromatherapy practitioner's reference library for blending are:

- ♠ *"The Complete Guide to Aromatherapy"* by Salvatore Battaglia.

- ♠ *"The Aromatherapy Workbook,"* by Marcel Lavabre.

- ♠ *"Aromatherapy Practitioner Reference Manual"* by Sylla Sheppard Hanger (two volumes).

- ♠ *"The Complete Book of Essential Oils and Aromatherapy"* by Valerie Ann Worwood.

Blending Techniques

Blending essential oils does not rely upon strict guidelines; instead, it requires knowledge of carrier oils and intuition that is gained only through familiarity with the oils and aromatherapy. As a beginner, it may be helpful to:

- ♠ Avoid blending more than three or four oils at a time until you gain considerable experience

- ♠ Ensure the blend's scent is pleasant to your patient/client (otherwise, the blend won't be used!)

- ♠ Review their intake form to confirm they do not have sensitivities/ allergies to the essential oils you wish to use

- ♠ Review their intake form to confirm they do not have medical conditions or are currently taking medications with contraindications to the essential oils used

- ♠ Ensure that your patient does not have an unpleasant memory associated with the oils you have selected

Quality is paramount in blending. When a lower quality lavender is used in the blend, it can start as a lovely scent. However, something doesn't smell right as the scent lingers in the air. This occurs when the stems and leaves are distilled along with the lavender flowers. The oil is considered a lower grade because the end product includes essential oil found in the stems and leaves instead of the flowers (also called adulteration). Only the highest quality of essential oils will result in effective, pleasant blends.

Top Notes

Using olfactory sense to identify the oils, as practiced with the kit and Personal Experience Handouts from Chapter 11, can you identify the first smell apparent when opening the vial of oil? A top note is apparent at the first fragrance (the first scent), and it dissipates quickly.

This occurs because the top note gives the first impression of the oil. The notes are sharp and penetrating – like peppermint – and can be refreshing and uplifting, and peppermint would be a top note. Essential oil top notes contain aldehydes and esters' biochemical constituents.

Typical top notes are bergamot, lemon, lime, and orange (citrus oils usually are top notes). Peppermint, thyme, cinnamon, clove, and lemongrass also can be considered top notes. While certain top notes can be used rather liberally, like lemon and bergamot, the sharpest ones – cinnamon and clove –require a much smaller amount. These sharp top notes should be blended in a smaller amount than a citrus top note. If too much cinnamon (or other sharp note) is used in your blend, it will overwhelm the blend's scent. The hot, caustic oils will last longer; therefore, less is needed when creating a blend (i.e., thyme, cinnamon, and clove).

Your top notes should constitute 20 to 40% of your blend. When using a 10ml bottle, then add 2 ml of the top note.

Middle Notes

Middle notes give the body to the blend. They are smooth, yet they have sharp edges with round corners, meaning the olfactory senses can initially detect the scent, then it disappears and can be re-detected with more prolonged exposure.

These oils are often referred to as blend enhancers; they enhance the scent of the blend and make it linger. The scent of the middle note lingers longer than the top note.

The top note is the first to be noticed, then the middle notes in the blend become obvious. Their fragrant qualities need to be appealing to the patient because they linger after the initial scent. Monoterpenes and alcohols are typically used as middle notes. These oils are generally harvested from leaves and herbs, including geranium, lavender, and marjoram. The middle notes usually form the majority of the blend: 40 to 80%.

Middle notes are also called the "heart" notes. As the center of the blend, these notes last the longest, revealing the warmth and fullness of the blend. They primarily influence digestion and the general metabolism of the body.

Base Notes

Base notes provide depth to the blend to hold and provide an anchor. The base notes are warm and rich and are normally pleasant. Most oils used as base notes have uses rooted in traditional rituals.

These oils have a strong effect on the mental, emotional, and spiritual planes and the astral body. When smelled from the bottle, the base notes may seem faint. But when applied to the skin, they react strongly and release scent and power. The oil needs to be released through a diffuser to capture those base notes, which typically include sandalwood, frankincense, myrrh, Vetiver, and patchouli. The plants for extraction are mostly found in woods, gums, and resins.

Base notes are long-lasting and act as fixatives. Fixatives reduce the top and middle notes' volatility rate and improve the blend's tenacity. A fixative is often grouped with essential oils to draw your blend into the skin and provide the body with constituents for healing. Whenever oils are applied to the skin, warm skin provides better absorption of the constituents. For base notes, 10 to 20% is ideal for creating your blend.

In *"The Aromatherapy Workbook,"* Marcel Levabre[1] writes about four categories that blending essential oils fall into:

1. **Blend equalizer:** These oils will soften sharp edges and fills the gaps so that the blend is in complete harmony and its vibrational frequency controls the intensity of the most active ingredient. The main purpose is to hold the blend together in perfect harmony.

2. **Blend modifier** (or personifier): These oils are generally the most intense fragrances and can greatly affect the overall fragrant quality of the blend, especially when used at a very small fraction of 1%. They also give your blend a "special kick" if its personality is not quite right or it seems flat or uninteresting.

3. **Blend enhancers:** Enhancers have a pleasant fragrance by themselves and have the personality to modify a blend with a personal touch without overpowering it when used in reasonable amounts.

4. **Natural extenders:** These oils are used with the most expensive and precious oils to make affordable blends without affecting the notes. When natural extenders are used, their fragrance should not be wasted, overpowered, or destroyed. Rather, they should be blended with essential oils that would be compatible.

Below are examples of essential oils that fall in each category:

Blend Equalizer	Blend Modifier	Blend Enhancer	Natural Extender
Rosewood	Clove	Bergamot	Petitgrain
Marjoram	Cinnamon	Cedarwood	Bergamot
Orange	Peppermint	Geranium	Geranium
Tangerine	Thyme	Clary sage	Benzoin

Blend Equalizer	Blend Modifier	Blend Enhancer	Natural Extender
Fir	Blue chamomile	Lavender	Peru balsam
Pine	Cistus	Lemon	Spruce
Champaca leaves	Patchouli	Palmarosa	
Petitgrain		Sandalwood	
		Ylang Ylang	
		Jasmine	
		Rose	
		Neroli	

When blending with precious oils such as neroli, rose, jasmine, or sandalwood, you want to find the essential oils that are the most compatible as possible from an olfactory point of view. I would suggest you do not mix eucalyptus with rose as an example because the eucalyptus would overpower the rose and waste the rose's beautiful scent.

The Psychological Aspect of Blending

The psychological aspect is important to designing the correct healing blend. Remember that when blending oils, it is necessary to be aware of the strong association between scent and memory.

The ability to build pictures and bridges using essential oils to associate images and feeling with fragrances can assist in understanding and aligning the constituents of the essential oils to our clients. For example, patchouli is an oriental market. Sandalwood is spiritual and meditative, and jasmine is sensual and erotic.

One need not be familiar with a particular fragrance for it to have an amazing influence. Pleasant odors will arouse happy and pleasant feelings unless those fragrances are associated with an unpleasant experience.

The ideal blend will create positive energy and interaction with the body on all levels – mental, emotional, psychological, and spiritual.

Practical Tips for Blending

A beautiful blend of essential oils should not break up into three stages when scented. If the blend is well balanced, the top note will contain some middle notes, the base note will retain some of the middle notes, and the changes during the evaporation process will be hardly noticeable. When you wave your hand over the blend or under your nose, you will feel, sense, and smell the essential oils working together – vibrating in unison. If the blend is not crafted well, it will fall apart and will smell each of the oils distinctly.

There is a scale developed by Louis Appell, *"Cosmetics, Fragrances, and Flavors: Their Formulation and Preparation,"* based on a scale from 1 to 10. The key to balance is achieving olfactory equilibrium, which occurs when two or more essential oils are in a mixture, and no single essential oil dominates the odor of the blend. For example, if you are making a blend with everlasting (helichrysum) and lavender, the respective odor intensities are 7 and 5. This means the odor of everlasting is stronger than that of lavender. As a result, mixing one drop of each will not produce a fragrance representing both essential oils and everlasting would dominate. Creating a beautiful blend may be necessary to mixing perhaps one drop of everlasting and three drops of lavender.

Odor Types

Blending can be created by odor types, using the essential oil scents to guide the combinations, in conjunction with the background of each client. While the descriptions are subjective, they provide useful, general guidance[1].

- ♠ Floral notes: Usually expensive and blend well with woody, fruity, sweet, and musty notes. It will be overwhelmed if used with camphoraceous notes.
- ♠ Fruity notes: Inexpensive and easy to blend. Do not blend well with woody notes and blend poorly with camphoraceous notes.
- ♠ Green notes: Blend well with any essential oil when used in small amounts.
- ♠ Herbaceous notes: Blend well with camphoraceous and woody notes. Use caution if combined with floral notes.

- ♠ Camphoraceous notes: Provide a "medicinal" scent to any blend, and it will ruin floral notes and does not blend well with fruity notes. Best used with herbaceous and woody notes.
- ♠ Spicy notes: They should be used in very small amounts (0.5% to 5%). They can add an interesting note to any blend; however, they can make or break a blend, so use them with caution.
- ♠ Earthy notes: Give depth and grounds any blend. Do not overuse; usually, 3% to 10% is sufficient.
- ♠ Woody notes: Bend well with any essential oils, creating warmth and giving the blend its heart-centeredness.

Some essential oils vary greatly in viscosity, with some having a thin consistency (lighter) while others are much thicker and heavier. These differences in consistency among essential oils can be described as their molecular weight or specific gravity. The thickness of an essential oil will determine the rate at which it comes out of the dropper. We reviewed this in Chapter 4, Chemistry, and Chapter 6, Safety, and it is also provided in GCMS data.

Proportions in Blending

Another important point about synergistic blends is ensuring the proportions are correct. Occasionally, preparing a larger volume than initially needed is necessary so that the smallest component oils can be incorporated into the whole in the right proportions. Diluted in a blend, you may have a component part that is only 0.001% of the whole, and yet that minuscule amount is integral to the whole[5].

Pipettes for measuring essential oil to create a blend comes in different sizes. Learning the sizes and consistency of the tools is important to create effective, balanced blends. Essential oils contain hundreds of chemical constituents and healing components. An entirely new compound is formed by blending two or more oils together, and the characteristics/effectiveness of the blend will change dramatically based on the proportions of each oil used.

Incorporating Quantum Healing in Blends

Once the essential oils, carrier oils, and enhancer lids are on tightly, the practitioner should gently roll the bottle between their palms and feel the vibrational frequency. To fully incorporate quantum healing, the practitioner should pause while holding the oil to intentionally seek the divine light of God and meditate on the love in this unique healing blend, incorporating mental, emotional, and spiritual strength and energy.

This intentionality during blending creates a type of synergy and connection between practitioner and patient, allowing this vortex of healing to take place. The mixture incorporates thought, intentions, and matter as the molecules are thoroughly blended.

As practitioner and client, sharing thoughts and their challenges through interviews and during the intake form creates mirror images, allowing the patient to trust and believe in your knowledge and ability to support them on their journey.

Handling essential oils is extremely important for quantum healing to take place. Quantum Healing differs from Western medicine in intentions and attention to the whole body rather than specific symptoms. Quantum healing takes place as support and balance of the many systems in the body rather than simply addressing a single issue. Underlying conditions, including mental and emotional challenges, are incorporated into a holistic approach to wellness and healing.

The quantum leap using essential oils will occur when the correct remedy, environment, and conditioning come together. The healing potential at that point is exponential. At the same time, blends created through frustration, anger, or inattention will not help the client/patient move forward with grace and ease. The intention and desire for healing need to be incorporated into the blend with the same intentionality as choosing the essential oils for the desired outcome.

Quantum Medicine

What is integrative quantum medicine? Its name is based on the physics theory that describes the similar movement of matter and energy. Quantum physics is the study of matter and energy at its most fundamental level, and a central tenet of quantum physics is that energy comes in indivisible packets called quanta. Quanta behave very differently from macroscopic matter: particles can behave like waves, and waves behave as though they are particles.

Quantum physics is relative to biology, the science of life. Physics is the foundation of sciences, yet many world views rely on Newtonian laws to describe matter and energy. *"Newtonian laws are used to describe expected actions of the physical world, and invisible quantum actions describing matter comprised of energy without absolutes are ignored. At the atomic level, matter does not even exist with certainty; it only exists as a tendency to exist*[3]*."*

Mahatma Gandhi's belief system supports the precepts of Quantum medicine. In his words, *"Your beliefs become your thoughts. Your thoughts become your words. Your words become your actions. Your actions become your habits. Your habits become your values. Your values become your destiny."*

Despite Western medicine's resistance to addressing the crucial role our minds play in our physical health, science readily confirms that physiological systems, primarily the body's skeletal musculature, are under the voluntary control of the conscious mind. Quantum healing and mental science research generally agree that only 5% of the brain controls our conscious mind. This leaves 95% of our brain operating subconsciously, which presents an incredible opportunity to change our thinking to move beyond programmed thought patterns that we follow without conscious decisions to a new pattern of choosing and healing that ultimately leads to physical and emotional peace and well-being.

When the conscious mind follows established historical patterns in behavior and choices, nothing changes. In order to produce real change, the conscious mind must begin the process of change within the subconscious through observation and proactive choices that fit a new pattern. The normal observer is often repeating life choices; therefore, the future and the past tend to follow similar patterns. Reactions, including choices and emotions, are often based on memory rather than current circumstances. Many individuals find it difficult to make new choices and changes because they are unable to move past familiar emotions, such as fear or anger, even when those emotions are detrimental to their lives. Quantum healing, from a cellular level to personal choices, changes our mindset to accept new possibilities, creating mental and body awareness. Once the body starts letting go of memories and emotions from the past, it starts to build new strength. When the human body is freed from the past, you can create never-ending change for a healthy mind, emotions, body, and attitude towards life.

Combined with changes over time, our body and mind are the basis of who we are—can change these building blocks of our perceived reality because quantum particles create waves of possibilities. When we release the negative/positive emotional charge from our life circumstances, we begin to live with wisdom and new opportunities. As a practitioner/healing, we use quantum healing to forge the body-mind connection and begin healing memory on a cellular level. Each cell in the human body contains not only the ability to remember but also the possibility of change and new pathways.

While the field is very new, research by geneticists/psychologists is demonstrating stress can be passed genetically through generations as part of epigenetics, which includes changes in organisms caused by gene expression modification rather than altering the genetic code. There is growing research that supports the idea that the effects of trauma can reverberate down the generations, based on studies of Union Army soldiers who were prisoners of war and their children/grandchildren, as well as studies of Holocaust survivors. If our cells have memory, then what controls the memory?

According to Dr. Bruce Lipton[3], the "magical membrane." The membrane is the cellular operation "gatekeeper," and the gatekeeper's role is controlling the "environment," which are the mechanisms by which the body translates environmental signals into behavior.

Our brain's ability to change its synaptic wiring by learning information and recording experiences is called neuroplasticity. Learning and changing allow humans to evolve our actions and modify our behavior to improve life in all aspects, including mental, emotional, spiritual, and physical. Neuro-rigidity would be the opposite, meaning only using our brain's prewired synaptic connections without learning from experience and creating new synaptic connections. Rigidity is to process the same thoughts, perform the same actions, and expect a different result.

Living with neuro-rigidity means thinking in the same box, i.e., living life according to past experiences without learning new patterns or being changed by new experiences. Neuroplasticity is thinking outside the box, learning new things, creating new experiences, and making new memories. At this point, the brain synapses are firing in unique patterns, and the neurons in the brain are making a new connection. The most straightforward functional unit of the nervous system is a neuron. Neurons possess the unique ability to store and communicate information, and learning from new experiences creates new synaptic connections. Remembering those experiences allows the brain to sustain these synaptic connections to make permanent new communication paths.
Dr. Joe Dispenza stated, "*Nerve cells that fire together, wire together. Meaning, when you create new learning and remembering, you are creating new thinking.*"[4]

- ♣ New experiences, when pursued and embraced, create a new thinking pattern by firing synaptic nerves. Without the stimulation from new experiences and ideas, nerves no longer fire together, and the new patterns and expansion are lost.

- ♣ Quantum medicine in this environment allows quantum healing to take place. Practicing quantum healing means becoming the observer of self and others to allow healing and optimization of our consciousness, brain, and thinking patterns. Consciousness mediates the action between mind and body. We, as humans, are caught between dualisms. Human consciousness is a nonlocal mediator between our mind and our body, where possibilities of every kind exist.

- ♣ Conscious intention works when intention becomes the freedom to choose possibilities. Once selected, possibilities become probabilities, which in turn become physical actualities according to the quantum possibility of thinking. Quantum consciousness exists where the freedom to choose is totally present. Thus, healing becomes a directive change from within the person, and consciousness is the mediator between physical and spiritual healing.

This paradigm shift encompasses alternative, complementary medicine to heal the four aspects of our entire body: mental, emotional, spiritual, and physical. As described in Chapter 4, Chemistry, all matter consists of base particles. Particles make atoms, atoms make molecules, molecules make cells, cells make up the brain, and the brain is responsible for consciousness and subjective experiences, including disease and healing. The experiences and patterns of our brains are connected to our health through our consciousness. The disease is not only caused by measurable physical challenges but also when the mind is trapped in neuro-rigidity. We must use neuroplasticity to think outside the box when looking to heal the entire body.

As a practitioner, clearing negative thoughts and personal concerns before handling essential oils allows positive energy from the oils, from the divine, and from the universe to flow through you to the remedy. Also important is developing readiness for a sacred moment and creating that consciousness of the essential oil blends as well as the entire healing on a quantum level.

When creating a blend for healing, keep that patient and their specific energy in mind; remember that quantum medicine is based on consciousness. Since consciousness is the ground for all existence, this thought process and energy go into a vibrational frequency of change. The practitioner should picture the resolution of the patient's challenges and/or issues on all levels of the healing: mental, emotional, spiritual, and physical, allowing for a tailored, supportive blend for healing the patient.

Infusing the essential oils with crystal energy can also be an option when looking for that existential aspect of healing. Prayer and reaching out for the blessings of Christ's consciousness is another aspect of combining quantum healing into an essential oil blend.

Blending is bringing all of the molecules together for the "connectedness" of mind, body, and spirit. Aromas can touch us and reconnect us mentally, emotionally, spiritually, and physically. When an aromatic molecule touches us, the molecule literally binds to one or multiple receptors in our body to influence and provide support and healing.

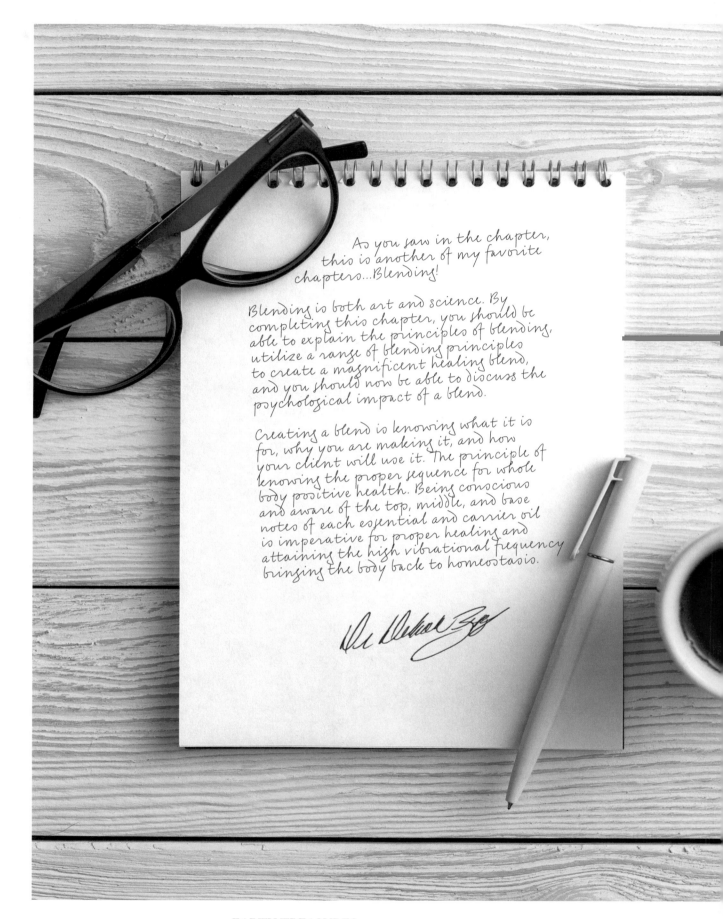

As you saw in the chapter, this is another of my favorite chapters...Blending!

Blending is both art and science. By completing this chapter, you should be able to explain the principles of blending, utilize a range of blending principles to create a magnificent healing blend, and you should now be able to discuss the psychological impact of a blend.

Creating a blend is knowing what it is for, why you are making it, and how your client will use it. The principle of knowing the proper sequence for whole body positive health. Being conscious and aware of the top, middle, and base notes of each essential and carrier oil is imperative for proper healing and attaining the high vibrational frequency bringing the body back to homeostasis.

Dr. Deborah Boss

Chapter Twelve References:

[1] Levabre, M., *Aromatherapy Workbook*. 1997, Healing Art Press, USA, page 111.

[2] Battaglia, S., *The Complete Guide to Aromatherapy, 2nd Edition, Perfect Potion Publisher*, page 360

[3] Lipton, B., MD, *The Biology of Belief*, Sounds True Publishing, page 86.

[4] Dispenza, J., *Breaking the Habit of Being Yourself*, page 33.

[5] Worwood, V.A., *The Complete Book of Essential Oils*, New World Library, page 5.

DELIVERY METHODS AND APPLICATIONS FOR ESSENTIAL OILS

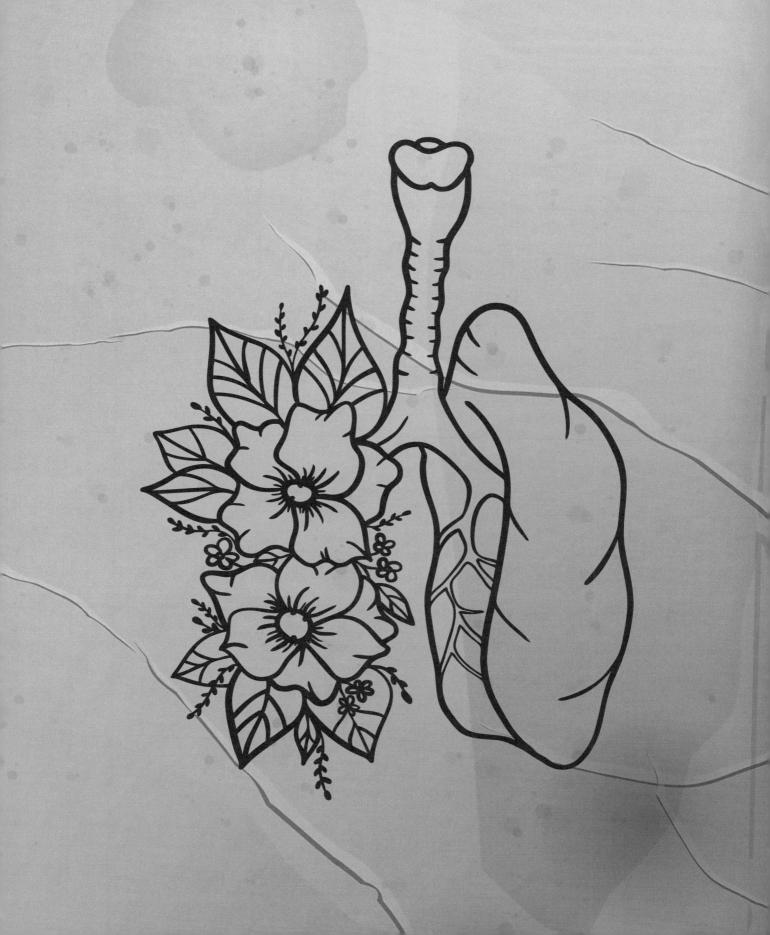

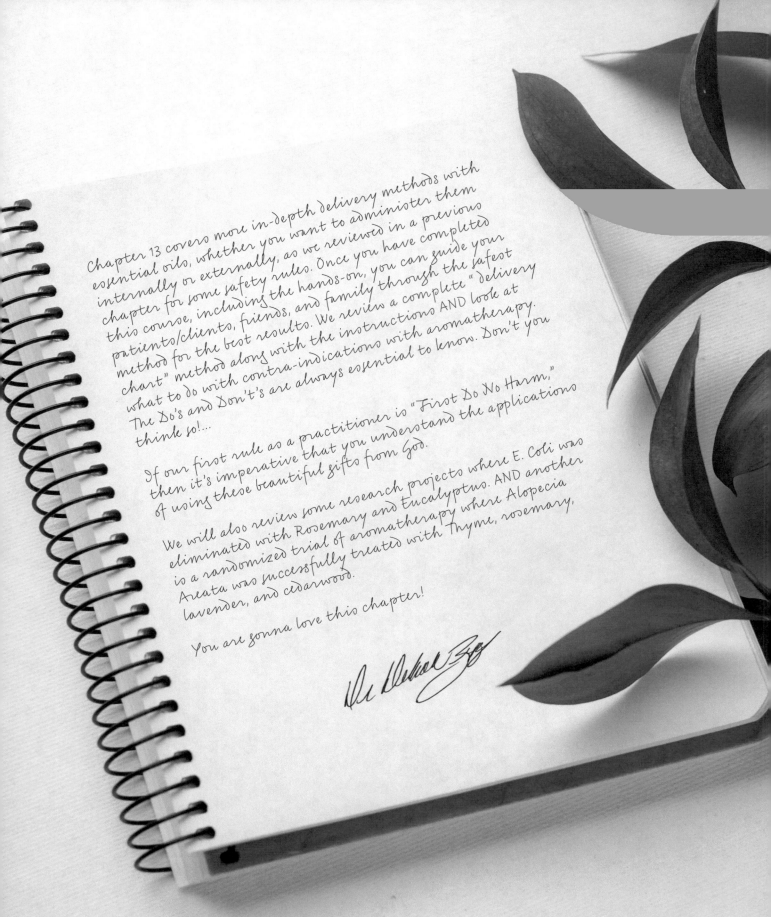

Chapter 13 covers more in-depth delivery methods with essential oils, whether you want to administer them internally or externally, as we reviewed in a previous chapter for some safety rules. Once you have completed this course, including the hands-on, you can guide your patients/clients, friends, and family through the safest method for the best results. We review a complete "delivery chart" method along with the instructions AND look at what to do with contra-indications with aromatherapy. The Do's and Don't's are always essential to know. Don't you think so!...

If our first rule as a practitioner is "First Do No Harm," then it's imperative that you understand the applications of using these beautiful gifts from God.

We will also review some research projects where E. Coli was eliminated with Rosemary and Eucalyptus. AND another is a randomized trial of aromatherapy where Alopecia Areata was successfully treated with Thyme, rosemary, lavender, and cedarwood.

You are gonna love this chapter!

EARTH TREASURES: A FOCUSED JOURNEY INTO THE FOUNDATIONS OF AROMATHERAPY

CHAPTER THIRTEEN:
DELIVERY METHODS AND APPLICATIONS FOR ESSENTIAL OILS

There are two delivery methods: internal and external, with several specific pathways for each one. While the pathways were mentioned in Chapter 3, Anatomy and Physiology in conjunction with body systems, this chapter provides more detail for choosing the most effective pathways and using them safely, correctly, and mindfully.

The information provided for chemical constituents of essential oils and the biochemistry of each, as well as the physical review in Chapter 11, describes the scent, touch, personality, and healing properties of each essential oil. By correctly identifying mental, emotional, or physical health issues, the knowledge of essential oils can be applied to select and support the well-being of yourself, friends, and family.

Internal Delivery Methods

As mentioned in the safety rules, internal usage should be solely under the guidance of a medical professional, such as an M.D. or clinical aromatherapist. A practitioner who is not a fully trained and licensed professional should seek to work in conjunction with a licensed professional. As a learning practitioner, it is prudent to use no more than three essential oils for internal use, and one or two is preferable.

Different formulas may be given at separate times of the day depending on the specific therapy required. Note that some oils have an excitatory effect that imbues energy and would not be appropriate to prescribe at night. Other oils can produce a calming, euphoric state and may not work well for a morning application. Regardless, all essential oils can provide support for healing if used according to the safety guidelines and the comprehension of their role in supporting the function of the systems of the human body.

General Rules

Safety first. Only non-toxic, non-irritant, non—sensitizing essential oils should be taken internally. The FDA provides up-to-date information on the Generally Regarded as Safe (GRAS) list. However, per the patient/ client's intake form, physical ailments and conditions may make an essential oil unsafe for that particular patient. Knowing and understanding the oils' chemical constituents and their effects on the body's systems will help you make the correct decision to provide safe, effective support and corrections for imbalances within the body.

Under the Tongue or the Roof of your Mouth

The essential oils must be diluted with either honey or carrier oil to ensure the fastest absorption into the bloodstream; otherwise, multiple applications can damage the tissue.

In the Form of Capsules

Typically 00, size capsules are made from gelatin. Always ensure the capsules do not contain microcrystalline or magnesium stearate, which are common ingredients in manufacturing capsules. Unfortunately, both ingredients affect the gut by blocking the absorption and communication of the cells. When using this application, also note that you should avoid highly irritant oils such as thyme, oregano, and cinnamon in the mouth because one drop undiluted can burn the mucous membrane tissue and potentially cause an ulcer. Always check the safety data sheet before using any essential oil to avoid injury. Unless specifically trained in the medical profession, aromatherapists cannot administer essential oils orally, nor should they diagnose, treat or prescribe. This responsibility is for qualified, licensed medical professionals.

When essential oils are taken internally, they are rapidly excreted through the urinary system bound with glucuronic acid, through the skin by sweat glands, and the lungs by exhalation. They usually pass through the body within 3 to 4 hours; however, some may dissipate as quickly as 0.5 hours (30 minutes).

Frequency

Both Dr. Jean Valnet, M.D. and Dr. Raphael D'Angelo, teaching medical professionals in this field, recommend that an oral regime include 2 to 4 drops, taken 3 to 4 times daily for a maximum of 4 weeks or less, depending on the toxicity of the essential oils [1][2]. The specific length of time will depend on the toxicity of the essential oils. Typically 2 to 3 weeks of this type of therapy is generally sufficient for acute conditions. Some ailments may only require 1 to 2 dosages if acute. Chronic cases should allow a minimum of 10 days between courses of treatment. Therefore, for approximately 2.5 weeks of therapy, allow ten days of rest. Please note the chronic toxicity (hepatic, nephritic) possibilities over long periods of treatment. Again, note that some essential oils cause mucus membrane irritation, and some are oral toxins.

Many professional aromatherapy associations do not endorse the internal ingestion of essential oils unless the aromatherapist has appropriate medical training. According to Salvatore Battaglia, oral administration does have many disadvantages[3]:

- Possibility of nausea
- Irritation of the gastrointestinal tract

- ♣ The metabolization of the essential oil by the liver
- ♣ Destruction of the essential oil constituents by stomach acidity or enzymes in the intestines

Rectal

Suppositories are a common method of essential oil administration by French medical doctors. The advantages of rectal application include:

- ♣ The essential oils can be administered in higher doses than orally for the challenges of acute infectious conditions, especially lower respiratory tract infections.
- ♣ The absence of the gastrointestinal tract and the essential oils and/or the liver eliminates the possibility of enzymes and acids breaking down the essential oil before.
- ♣ It allows faster absorption into the body.
- ♣ Reduced possible liver challenges especially oils containing phenols (in order to excrete the phenols, they must be converted into sulfonates, which may cause damage to the liver).
- ♣ Suppositories are easier to administer safely than oral ingestion, without the concerns of capsule ingredients.

External Delivery Methods

Chapter 3 describes skin and pathway for essential oil application. However, very little research exists on the effects of essential oils externally. Whole essential oils may not be fully absorbed into the skin and enter the blood stream through this pathway. However, skin application is beneficial to the mental state (relaxation) and may allow additional benefits with massage essential oil therapies to treat the entire body. Skin treatments affect the external layers and can support conditions and ailments that occur on those layers as well as enhancing healing with the olfactory senses.

Essential oil antimicrobial and anti-inflammatory properties, along with many other medicinal properties, have proven excellent for supporting minor ailments. The beneficial mental effects from using a pleasing fragrance are both immediate and lasting.

Chart for delivery method. The chart below was compiled by Sylla Sheppard-Hanger in "*The Aromatherapy Practitioner Reference Manual.*" This chart can be used as a starting point to expand over time with your experience and knowledge.

Application Method	Number of Drops	Amount of Carrier Oil
Massage oil	15 25-30 drops 40-60 drops	30 ml. (1 oz) carrier 60 ml 120 ml carrier
Massage (local use)	25-30 drops	30 ml (1 oz) carrier
Topical use (acute or acupressure)	50-60 drops	30 ml (1 oz) carrier
Neat (undiluted)	1-2 drops	Nonirritating oils, only on stings, pimples (lavender, tea tree, rosewood, thyme linalool, Ravensara, etc.)
Facial oil	25 drops	30 ml (1 oz) carrier
Facial steam	5-7 drops	Per cups of water (or in steamer)
Hair/scalp oil	25 drops	30 ml carrier oil
Inhalation	Start with 2-3 and work up to 5-7 drops	Bowl of hot water, tower over the head, inhale. Or use micro diffuser, inhale until you stop smelling oil. 15-20 minutes. Repeat every 3-4 hours. *
Micro diffusion	5-10 drops	Inhale near the glass nebulizer (glass should be type with beak, producing millions of ionized particles in a barely visible steam
Humidifiers	3-10 drops	Add to water, repeat after a few hours or run over night
Bath	5-15 drops	Add to milk/egg yolk/Epsom salts and/or hydrogen peroxide then add warm water, swish *
Compress	4-6 drops	Bowl of warm water, skim surface with cloth, wring, apply over area, repeat when cool
Water spray (Spritzer)	8-10 drops Face 30-40 drops Body 80-100 drops per room	Per 120 ml (4 oz) distilled water, shake, spray; use for facial toner, body wrap, room spray

Application Method	Number of Drops	Amount of Carrier Oil
Douche	10-40 drops	Per pint of warm water, shake before using. Add apple cider vinegar to help maintain Ph balance
Body wrap	Make spritzer above	Spay towel, wrap body, wrap with plastic sheet, blanket, relax 20 min.
Jacuzzi	3 drops per gallon	Add to water *
Sauna	1-2 drops per cup of water	Use eucalyptus, tea tree, pine oils; shake and throw on heat source as usual.
Shower	4-8 drops	After shower, apply to washcloth, rub over body briskly
Bath Salts	5-8 drops per cup	Use equal parts: Epsom salts (magnesium sulfate), sea salt (and/or baking soda); rub on clean wet skin for "salt glow" or dissolve in water for bath.
Dry brush	1-3 drops	Apply to natural bristle brush, brush extremities in direction of the heart, (before or after shower, bath.
Floral waters, hydrolat, distillate	Byproduct of essential oil steam distillation	Contains water soluble compounds, carboxylic acids, terpenes, tannings, flavonoids, and sesquiterpene alcohols, cooling anti-inflammatory agents. Use as toners, for compresses, drink as tea, (2 tbsp in 8oz mineral water)
Suppositories	5-10 drops in 15 ml carrier oil	Preblend; inject ¼ pipette rectally for serious infection (flu, bronchitis, stomach infection)

(Sheppard-Hanger)[4]

Note: (*) As a safety rule, oil and water don't mix. Contraindications with Massage Aromatherapy.

Just because essential oils can be purchased at grocery stores and they are found in many products, does not prove the oils are safe for use in all situations. When receiving or performing any essential oil therapy, even informally with family, friends, or providing advice, the following safety cautions apply:

- **Postoperative care.** Always ask permission from client, client's doctor or surgeon before massaging, especially after major surgery (if you are using a diffuser). Some essential oils might have contraindications with the prescriptions.
- **Varicose veins.** Massage the essential oils extremely light over these areas and always upward strokes only. Never downward.
- **Heart conditions.** If the client has a history of heart attack, angina or stroke, apply essential oils to reflex points (hands and feet) and perhaps the back (gently) to help the circulation. Again, Note the potential for contraindications with prescriptions.
- **Infectious diseases.** Do not ever massage any topical infections; instead, use compresses and diffusers for broken skin and/or wounds. Floral waters/hydrosols can also be effective in spritzer on skin and perhaps for bedsores. (compress works great here as well). Chest and back massage can provide effective relief for respiratory infections such as bronchitis, sore throat, or chest infection.
- **Cancer.** More hospitals are recognizing the effective support of essentials oils with massage for cancer patients to help alleviate symptoms from chemotherapy or radiation therapy. Many massage schools teach this specific type of massage to help cancer patients. However, if you are not a massage therapist, you can always help with other methods such as diffuser, reflexology, as well as providing hydrolats. Again, confirm potential contraindications as well as the dangerous or lethal dosages before any application.
- **Inflamed joints.** Essential oil therapy is useful for imbalances in the body such as arthritis through massage and/or applying essential oils directly over the area, gently. If the patient's pain level will not allow direct touch, the application can include a bath or compress using the correct and safe oils. Applying oils or massaging directly over the painful joints may cause initial pain but doing so can prove beneficial to circulation if the patient can endure.
- **Fractures and large areas of scars.** Do not massage large area of scars for at least two months post surgery. Hydrosols, compresses, or a diffuser may be used to minimize the scarring and bring calm. The oils

may also allow better sleep and healing by relaxing the body and mind. For fractures, oils can also be used to induce and enhance sleep to heal the body and reduce pain.

Spinal Application/Castor Oil Pack

Chapter 3, Lesson 7 provided a description of the spine and the challenges if the related systems, organs, and/or vertebrae are not in harmony.

Please keep the charts from Chapter 3 available when looking for the root causes of the imbalances within the body. When working with the spine, compresses can provide effective remedies. As a massage therapist, applying 1 to 2 drops directly to the spine and gently massaging the application area will provide immediate support. Another effective application is to apply the essential oils to the correct location on the back, place a warm towel over the area, and then apply heat (such as a hot water bottle). This application pushes the essential oils deeper into the body, allowing the body to relax and absorb the medicinal properties.

The castor oil pack is a traditional aromatic medicine therapy. Use ½ yard of 100% cotton flannel or 100% natural color wool. (enough fabric to create a four-ply of fabric that to covers the area). Completely saturate the layers of fabric (but not dripping). Place the oil-saturated flannel directly on the skin and cover with a piece of plastic such as a plastic bag or plastic wrap. Apply heat using a hot water bottle, heating pad, or hot towel over the plastic. Leave in place for a minimum of 90 minutes. A castor oil pack can be placed on the following body regions:

- Right of the abdomen to stimulate and detoxify liver
- Inflamed and swollen joints, bursitis and muscle strains
- Abdomen to relieve constipation and other digestive disorders
- Lower abdomen for menstrual irregularities and uterine and ovarian cysts.

Physiological effects of castor oils packs include:
- Improves the elimination in the gastrointestinal and genito-urinary tract
- Balances acid secretions in the stomach
- Stimulates peristalsis and improves assimilation in the gastrointestinal tract
- Stimulates liver, pancreas, and gall bladder secretions
- Maintains the mucous membrane lining
- Improves coordination of the functions of major organs, glands, and systems
- Helps control inflammation
- Stimulates the nervous system

♣ Improves lymphatic circulation (waste removal)

♣ Draws acids and infections out of the body.

Do not reuse the cloth! It has pulled toxins from the body and washing does not remove them.

	Organ Connection	Potential Support and Healing Oil
C 1	Head, optical nerve, brain	*7th Energy Center Blend* sandalwood, frankincense rosewood basil
C 2	Eyes, tongue, ears, sinuses	*6th Energy Center Blend* Cedarwood atlas, peppermint rosemary (1,8 cineol)
C 3	Ears, teeth, facial nerves	*5th Energy Center Blend* clove, Roman chamomile, spearmint, peppermint, Eucalyptus radiata
C 4	Nose, mouth, lips, ears, mandibular joint, throat	*5th Energy Center Blend* lavender, geranium frankincense, rose otto, cinnamon, Eucalyptus globulus
C 5	Cervical muscles, throat, neck	*5th Energy Center Blend* sandalwood, spikenard, tea tree, clary sage, thyme (red)
C 6	Acromioclavicular joint, shoulder, tonsils, neck	*5th Energy Center Blend* clove, cinnamon, geranium, tea tree
C 7	Thyroid gland, elbow, sternoclavicular joint	*5th Energy Center Blend* peppermint, sweet marjoram, ylang ylang, jasmine
Th1	Shoulder, wrist, hand, neck, lower arm, fingers	*4th Energy Center Blend* bergamot, sandalwood, Roman chamomile, valerian
Th2	Heart, blood vessels, chest	*4th Energy Center Blend* benzoin, lime, melissa, sandalwood, fennel, cypress, mandarin, bergamot
Th3	Lung, skin, breasts, chest, mammary gland	*4th Energy Center* Virginian cedarwood, lemon, rose otto, sweet fennel, Australian sandalwood
Th4	Gallbladder, tendons, ligaments	*3rd Energy Center Blend* black pepper, cinnamon, lemon, thyme (ct linalool)

	Organ Connection	Potential Support and Healing Oil
Th5	Liver, circulatory system, immune system, tendons, ligaments	*3rd Energy Center Blend* citronella, sweet fennel, ylang ylang, tea tree, cedarwood atlas, rosemary verbenone
Th6	Stomach, muscles, pancreas	*3rd Energy Center Blend* ginger, lemon, peppermint, oregano
Th7	Duodenum, stomach, pancreas, muscles	*3rd Energy Center Blend* niaouli, cinnamon, helichrysum, peppermint
Th8	Spleen, blood, muscles	*3rd Energy Center Blend* niaouli, cinnamon, helichrysum, peppermint, thyme (chemotype thujanol-4), nutmeg
Th9	Adrenal gland	*2nd Energy Center Blend* clary sage, orange, rose otto, myrrh, lavender, marjoram
Th10	Kidney, bones	*2nd Energy Center Blend* neroli, grapefruit, juniper berry, lavender
Th11	Skin, kidney, urinary track, bones	*2nd Energy Center Blend* rose otto, clary sage, jasmine, myrrh
Th12	Small intestine, ovary, testicles, blood vessels, circulation	*2nd Energy Center Blend* orange, geranium, cypress, angelica root
L 1	Large intestine, skin	*1st Energy Center Blend* cardamom, cedarwood atlas, peppermint, eucalyptus, lemon, basil
L 2	Large bowel, appendix skin	*1st Energy Center Blend* spikenard, juniper berry, clary sage
L 3	Bladder, uterus, prostate, knee	*1st Energy Center Blend* ginger, cedarwood atlas, peppermint, rose damask, frankincense
L 4	Sigmoid, sciatic nerve, prostate	*1st Energy Center Blend* peppermint, cardamom, myrrh, sandalwood
L 5	Rectum	*1st Energy Center Blend* mandarin, cypress, rosemary (camphor or 1,8 cineol)
SI	Sacrum, legs, hip, sciatic nerve, crest, buttock, genital organs	*1st Energy Center Blend* peppermint, Eucalyptus radiata, clove, geranium, lavender
SI	Coccyx, Anus	*1st Energy Center Blend* ginger, cinnamon, myrrh, cajeput, cedarwood atlas, lemon, thyme (red)

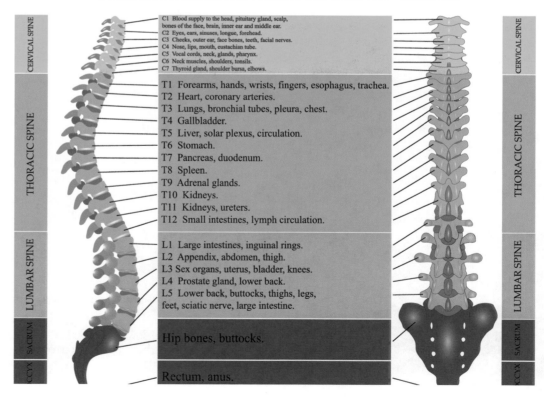

SAHASRARA		CROWN CHAKRA Spirituality
AJNA		THIRD EYE CHAKRA Awareness
VISHUDDHA		THROAT CHAKRA Communication
ANAHATA		HEART CHAKRA Love • Healing
MANIPURA		SOLAR PLEXUS CHAKRA Wisdom • Power
SVADHISHTHANA		SACRAL CHAKRA Sexuality • Creativity
MULADHARA		ROOT CHAKRA Basic trust

VERTEBRA FRONT AND SIDE

CERVICAL SPINE

C1 Blood supply to the head, pituitary gland, scalp, bones of the face, brain, inner ear and middle ear.
C2 Eyes, ears, sinuses, tongue, forehead.
C3 Cheeks, outer ear, face bones, teeth, facial nerves.
C4 Nose, lips, mouth, eustachian tube.
C5 Vocal cords, neck, glands, pharynx.
C6 Neck muscles, shoulders, tonsils.
C7 Thyroid gland, shoulder bursa, elbows.

THORACIC SPINE

T1 Forearms, hands, wrists, fingers, esophagus, trachea.
T2 Heart, coronary arteries.
T3 Lungs, bronchial tubes, pleura, chest.
T4 Gallbladder.
T5 Liver, solar plexus, circulation.
T6 Stomach.
T7 Pancreas, duodenum.
T8 Spleen.
T9 Adrenal glands.
T10 Kidneys.
T11 Kidneys, ureters.
T12 Small intestines, lymph circulation.

LUMBAR SPINE

L1 Large intestines, inguinal rings.
L2 Appendix, abdomen, thigh.
L3 Sex organs, uterus, bladder, knees.
L4 Prostate gland, lower back.
L5 Lower back, buttocks, thighs, legs, feet, sciatic nerve, large intestine.

SACRUM

Hip bones, buttocks.

COCCYX

Rectum, anus.

The spine holds our entire body upright. It connects our entire body physically, as well as supporting the mental, emotional, and spiritual well-being. Understanding these connections is important when using essential oils on the spine and back areas.

Diffusing Essential Oils

Diffusers have become commonplace and can be found on shelves in most grocery and department store, claiming to provide numerous benefits with extra features (rock salt, lights, and music). Knowing that the olfactory system provides the best pathway for delivery, a diffuser should be a standard in home and office. Many different types exist with positives and perhaps negatives for each:

- **Water diffusers.** Water diffusers provide 36 hours and radiate 400 square feet. (localized application). In this instance, oil and water do mix due to the small ionization being applied to the oils to break down into smaller molecules to be dispersed. Unless thoroughly cleaned the residue from oils will linger. Essential oils also degrade plastic, so a plastic diffuser should be cleaned regularly with vinegar or rubbing alcohol.
- **Micro diffusers.** While expensive, these diffusers provide excellent support for lung and sinus challenges. Nebulizers are used in the medical field to deliver asthma and lung medications. Micro diffusers have a glass tube while nebulizers have a mask that covers the mouth and nose for effective, direct delivery.
- **Candle Diffusers.** These are very pretty and can bring a lovely atmosphere, however, heat destroys the medicinal properties of the essential oils.
- **Light bulb and Essential Oil Dispenser.** While safer than the candle diffuser (normally, these are low heat), the heat still destroys the properties of the essential oil.
- **Humidifiers.** Great source to disperse the essential oils to provide both support from the oil and hydration for illnesses. However, essential oils degrade plastic, wood, etc., so the humidifier should be cleaned regularly with vinegar (soak for 10 to 15 minutes) or rubbing alcohol.
- **Candles.** When using candles for therapy, identification of the exact essential oils (and any other chemical constituents) is nearly impossible unless making them yourself. Again, heat destroys the biochemical constituents (thus, eliminating medicinal therapy).
- **Ceramic Lightbulb Rings/Stones.** These diffusers are small, convenient, and easy to use. The light bulb ring style fits most bulbs, although the essential oil should be applied to the ring before placing onto light bulb. Essential oil stones can be placed strategically around the room, and as the stone reaches the room temperature, the essential oil is released.

♠ **Cotton Balls.** This method is simple, quick, easy, and very economical. Teachers often use this method for classrooms when an electric diffuser is not allowed. By applying some essential oils on cotton balls and placing around the room, the mental and emotional support provides a more attentive and healthier atmosphere for education. Cotton balls can be stored in your vehicle and in your purse for quick application and easy cleanup

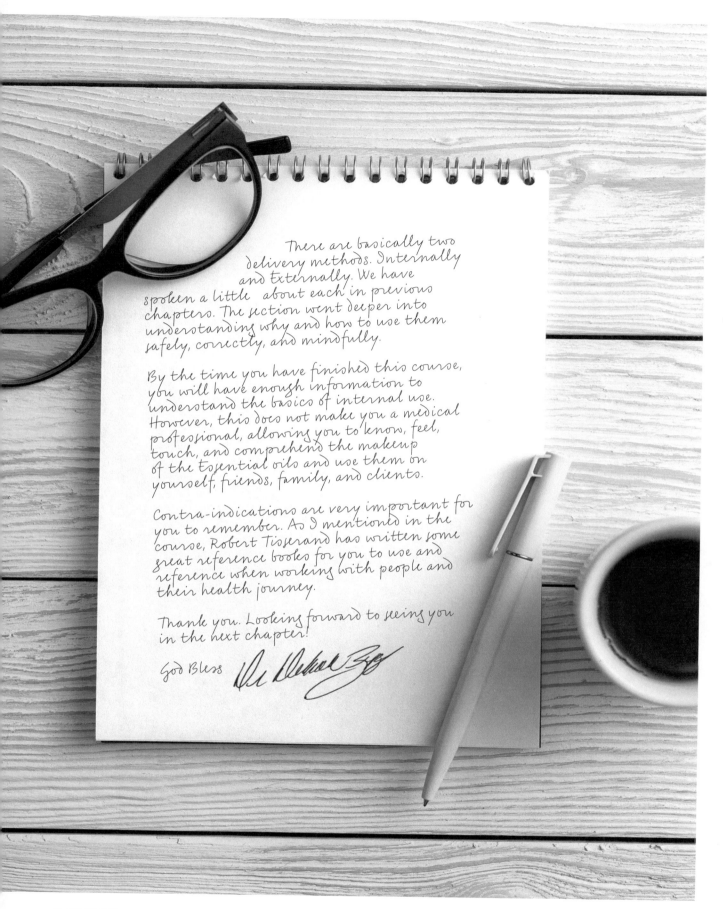

There are basically two delivery methods. Internally and Externally. We have spoken a little about each in previous chapters. The section went deeper into understanding why and how to use them safely, correctly, and mindfully.

By the time you have finished this course, you will have enough information to understand the basics of internal use. However, this does not make you a medical professional, allowing you to know, feel, touch, and comprehend the makeup of the Essential oils and use them on yourself, friends, family, and clients.

Contra-indications are very important for you to remember. As I mentioned in the course, Robert Tisserand has written some great reference books for you to use and reference when working with people and their health journey.

Thank you. Looking forward to seeing you in the next chapter!

God Bless

Chapter Thirteen References:

[1] Valnet, J., M.D., *The Practice of Aromatherapy*, page 215.

[2] D'Angelo, R., M.D., *Medical Aromatherapy, Level II Class,* Alliance of International Aromatherapist (AIA) accredited, 2006.

Author's Note: *Dr. Raphael J.d'Angelo received his medical degree from University of Oklahoma College of Medicine in 1976.He has authored numerous health articles, chapters for medical textbooks and patient education publications. He is an active researcher in infectious diseases, he is a respected leader in the natural treatment of infectious conditions. Dr. D'Angelo may be reached at www. parawellnessresearch.com) His courses were given in his medical practice physical office at 18121-C. East Hampden Avenue #123, Aurora Colorado 80013.*

[3] Battaglia, S,. *"The Complete Guide to Aromatherapy."* 2nd edition, page 373.

[4] Sheppard-Hanger, S., *The Aromatherapy Practitioner Reference Manual,* Atlantic Institute of Aromatherapy, 1995, page 6.

FROM THE FIELD: Bridget Kelley, President of Kelly Pure Essential Oils

We all try to achieve harmony within ourselves and to help the people around us. Dr. Zepf's Clinical Therapy Practitioner Certification is <u>the</u> quintessential Level 3 Aromatherapy course that you have been looking for. In it, she addresses the holistic healing aspect that is missing in our everyday life. It is the lack of treating the whole person that keeps us from the harmony that leads us to a healthy life. Quantum medicine: a means to examine the body from health to sickness, is an intrinsic part of the curriculum, which ultimately aids us in being healthy and whole. You will have interactive learning, along with hours of direct, one-on-one instruction – unlike any other online certification. Dr. Zepf's extensive knowledge of essential oils is the foundation of this course. She has also combined all her knowledge of the modalities she practices and has included them to enhance your all-around knowledge of essential oils and their uses. Upon completion, you will have gained a greater understanding of the safe, effective, and positive use of essential oils. Whether you use essential oils for your personal use, business practice or in a clinical setting, you will do so with greater confidence and assurance.

I have known and worked with Dr. Zepf for over 10 years. We met at the Alliance of International Aromatherapists (AIA) annual Aromatherapy Conference in Chicago. Her fun, upbeat and positive demeanor was an instant attraction. Her love for the oils is very apparent and contagious. From there we both sat on the Board of Directors for AIA and served on their Annual Conference committee for numerous years. Currently, as a supplier of essential oils, we collaborate on industry news, essential oil supply and demand issues, reviewing GC/MS reports, staying up to date on the CITES list and sharing our current favorite essential oil with love and laughter.

As the increasing consumer awareness of wanting natural and organic options in their health care, the consumer is shifting their focus to essential oils as a means to improve their wellness plan. The industry is expected to grow up to 46.4% in the next 8 years. The amount of information that is available to the public is vast and you will need to be able to discern the accuracy and validity of this information for the safety of yourself and those that you serve. By completing this course to be accredited as a Professional Clinical Aroma Therapy Practitioner, you will gain the expertise to not only be knowledgeable about essential oils but also the voice of reason within your community.

"Health is a state of complete harmony of the body, mind and spirit. When one is free from physical disabilities and mental distractions, the gates of the soul open."

B.K.S Lyengar

Bridget Kelley
President of Kelley Pure Essential Oils
Registered Aromatherapist
Community Herbalist, Naturalist, Master Gardener
Past President of Alliance of International Aromatherapists
Former Oncology Massage Therapist
New Richmond, WI
August 2022

THE BUSINESS END: CREATING A PROFESSIONAL BUSINESS PRACTICE

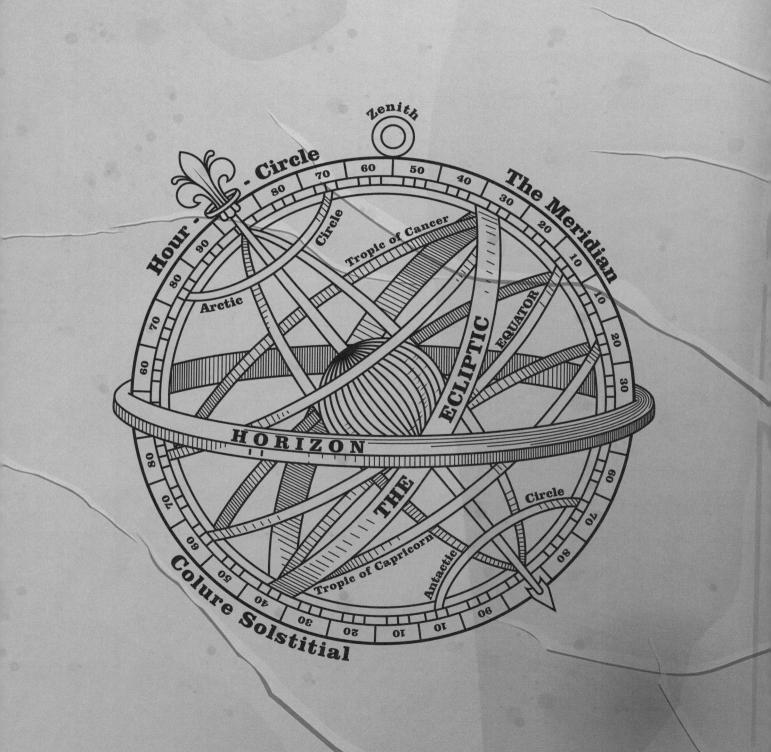

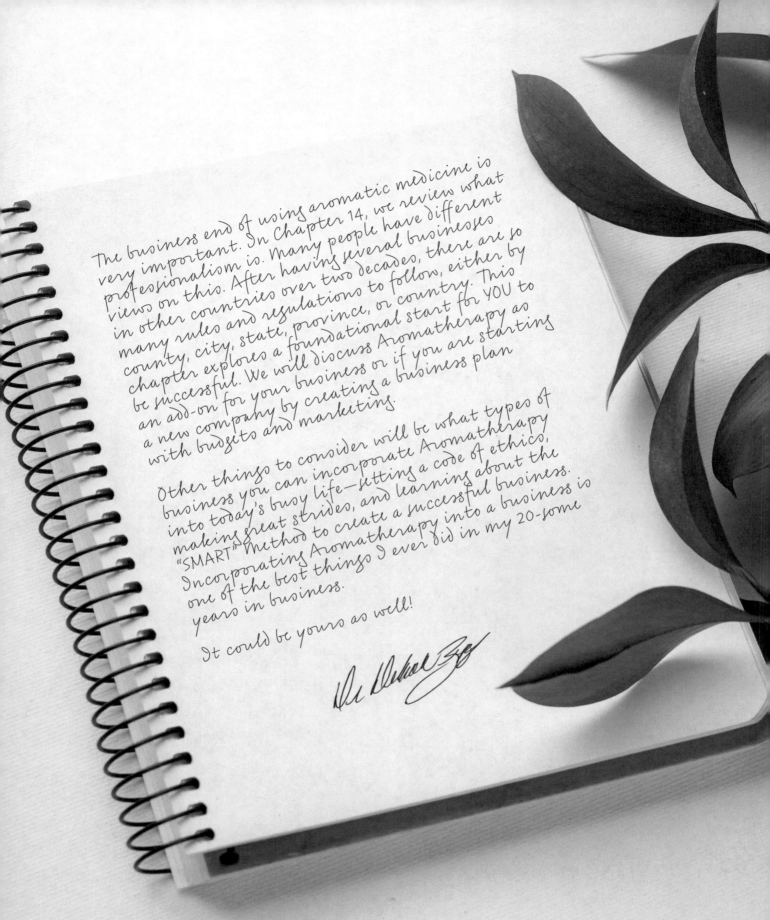

The business end of using aromatic medicine is very important. In Chapter 14, we review what professionalism is. Many people have different views on this. After having several businesses in other countries over two decades, there are so many rules and regulations to follow, either by country, city, state, province, or country. This chapter explores a foundational start for YOU to be successful. We will discuss Aromatherapy as an add-on for your business or if you are starting a new company by creating a business plan with budgets and marketing.

Other things to consider will be what types of business you can incorporate Aromatherapy into today's busy life—setting a code of ethics, making great strides, and learning about the "SMART" method to create a successful business. Incorporating Aromatherapy into a business is one of the best things I ever did in my 20-some years in business.

It could be yours as well!

Dr. Deborah Bey

CHAPTER FOURTEEN:
THE BUSINESS END: CREATING A PROFESSIONAL BUSINESS PRACTICE

Starting a successful business means building a solid foundation that includes fit-for-purpose marketing, finances, and products tailored to meet specific business needs. Without a great foundation, any business will crumble. According to the U.S. Bureau of Labor Statistics (2019), approximately 20% of new businesses fail within the first two years, 45% within the first five years, and 65% within the first ten years. Only 25% of new businesses will survive 15 years or more. The most common reasons for these failures include lack of business experience, lack of business planning, and lack of cash flow planning.

Understanding essential oils and aromatherapy for healing is the first step to developing a successful business or practice. Developing business skills is necessary to operate a successful aromatherapy practice, whether providing simple aromatherapy or adding services as a therapy.

From state practice registration to collecting required sales tax, medical licensing and practicing laws are stringent and vary according to city, state, county, and country. Every practice must comply with all applicable laws, and ensuring compliance will require research of local, state, and federal statutes to determine and meet all necessary requirements.

Business Incorporation and Planning

Incorporation
Businesses may operate as sole proprietors, partnerships, corporations, or limited liability corporations. Each requires a federal (and sometimes state) incorporation to receive an Employer Identification Number (EIN). An EIN, also known as a Federal Tax Identification Number, is used to identify a business entity. Businesses can apply online for an EIN as a free service offered by the Internal Revenue Service. First, determine if your state requires a number or charter, then use that identification for the federal application.

Planning
Connecting with other practitioners who have established successful businesses (or small business owners, whether in aromatherapy or other industries) can be key to successful business planning. Finding a mentor with proven success can be the best resource for positive, helpful feedback in each process step.

Building a successful business must include a written plan that addresses the main steps for a start-up. Putting the plan on paper provides a solid outline of action steps and a plan that can be shared with a mentor for suggestions and advice. It is also necessary to have a written plan when approaching a financial institution or friend for investment.

The plan should:

- ♠ Develop monthly projections for the first year and include at least three years
- ♠ Estimate sales, including total sales and product breakdown
- ♠ Define expenses such as inventory, supplies, shipping costs, salaries
- ♠ If selling retail, include obtaining a state retail sales tax license
- ♠ If needed, have obtained credit card merchant services (understand that credit card companies charge as much as 2.5%)
- ♠ Include monthly interest payments if borrowing money
- ♠ Include rent costs as applicable; working from home means charging the company rent for using space and utilities
- ♠ Include insurance costs

Show profit with your plan using a balance sheet; if it doesn't show any profit, then change the plan.

Making a plan includes general and specific knowledge of business operations. Similar to understanding the personality and chemical constituents of each essential oil, each business owner must understand the general and specific information of aromatherapy business and marketing:

Know your Market. What essential oils are most popular and will sell quickly? Controlling initial costs using popular essential oils will provide better cash flow control. Also, develop an advertising plan for the identified audience (communications should describe the products/services and demonstrate effectiveness for wellbeing and overall support).

Know your Product. Lavender has over 39 different species with five essential oil types, which vary in price and quality. Most people will not know the difference, but the practitioner should be an expert on essential oil properties, blends, notes, and costs. The practitioner should also be able to communicate to clients, patients, and customers what essential oils are in stock and how these support ailments and overall wellbeing.

Know your Inventory. Inventory is an investment in a product, and if it does not sell immediately, then that cost must be carried out until it does. Managing inventory is critical to a successful business; knowing what products are needed, how many are stocked, how much it costs to carry that stock, and how often it sells. In a computerized inventory system or regular, the physical count is invaluable for replacing products as they sell. QuickBooks® software is an effective tool to keep inventory levels and sales accurate and manage payments and invoices.

Know Cost/Quality/Pricing. Research carefully to find a good supplier offering a reasonable price, quality, and reliable shipment service. An excellent reputation can be destroyed in a second through one bad product or inability to get the product in a reasonable time. Suppliers are a partner to success.

Know your Total Costs. The total cost of each product sold includes:
- Wholesale price plus shipping
- Advertising costs
- Marketing costs
- Special labeling costs, etc.

The fair market price and any competitor's sale price should be used to determine the appropriate price for each product.

Additional New Business Plan Requirements

Sales

Alongside knowledge and skills with essential oils, serving as a sales representative is key to success. Connecting potential customers with the proper essential oil support is foundational to both immediate sales and developing a long-term customer base. Remember, the nature of essential oil is to provide alignment and support over time, and so a practical approach to sales is developing long-term relationships.

Also, for the most effective use of time and money, selling one item for $40 is better than $1 item to 40 customers, so consider selling sets, blends, and things that have added value (e.g., soaps with essential oils in them). Free samples are only free to the customer, so they should produce profits from the time and energy invested, such as new clients or increased business.

Steps for Success
1. **Write a complete business plan.** Writing the plan in detail creates more of a commitment and allows scrutiny of others. Asking for guidance from a successful small business owner can help to identify weaknesses in the plan.

2. **Use your finances wisely.** Develop savings for investment in your own business and start small. Borrowing money from other sources can be helpful before a positive cash flow, but interest and payments will limit your ability to be profitable.

3. **Become an expert salesperson.** Know your product and your business. With your specialized knowledge of essential oils and the specific healing/helping chemical properties, you should be able to ascertain what support each customer needs and guide them to appropriate choices and investments.

4. **Research for an essential oil supplier.** Find the most reliable, cost-effective supplier who provides good quality products and build a long-term relationship. Locate more than one supplier to ensure product availability.

5. **Research your market.** Develop solid research for what products people buy and fair market price. Develop a target market with detailed information on where your target market spends their money, such as online purchases, local gift shops, or local medical offices.

6. **Define detailed costs for all business supplies.** Costs should include products, initial investments in hardware and software for product inventory, accounting, marketing, utilities, rent, and salaries (if you intend to hire employees).

7. **Manage your inventory closely.** Essential oils have a limited shelf life, so only needed supplies should be kept on hand (never overstock). Ensure suppliers can ship products on a timely basis.

8. **Become creative in product development.** Develop essential oil kits (such as blends for specific ailments or holidays, essential oil sets, and value-added products such as candles or kinds of butter with essential oils).

In a business we must follow not only our own code of ethics but also sanitary practices for our business. Again, this makes us professional, ethical, and mindful of ourselves and other people. Of course, you understand the essential oil rules for using these precious gifts from God, and we want to ensure that the clients feel safe and trusts in you.

Business Alignments to Define:
- Type of business services
- Importer/supplier
- Practitioner
- Multi-level marketing rep
- Essential oil practitioner
- Counselor
- Educator
- Massage therapist
- Reflexologist

Supplies and Equipment Needed:
- Essential oils
- Carrier oils
- Ointment/creams
- Bottles – different sizes, different applications
- Labels
- Massage tables
- Pipettes
- Hydrolats/hydrosol

Developing Your Personal Path Forward

Starting any business means following your dream, heart, joy, and passion. Your changes in mindset and life lessons through personal coaching and understanding of your gifts will help align goals with life choices, moving from untrained handler/practitioner and user to practical clinical aromatherapist to teacher.

Life is all about learning and yearning. Every person is both a physical and a spiritual being, living an experience that is both spiritual and physical. Sharing the healing and wellbeing of essential oils allows the practitioner to combine these experiences.

Marguerite Ham has over 30 years of experience in training, coaching, leadership development, conferences, and professional retreats with organizations nationwide. She is a Certified DISC Practitioner and Partner, Human Capital Coach, and Grief and Loss Coach. Marguerite believes the answers you seek lie within you, and through artful listening and coaching, those answers are revealed, allowing you to align your actions with your values. Living your values is the key to deep fulfillment and joy at work and home. In addition, she uses horses in coaching and leadership training to allow experiential growth. Marguerite has certifications in Equine-Assisted Psychotherapy, Equine-Assisted learning, Equine-Facilitated Coaching, and Horse Strong Coaching.

Working together to apply Marguerite's knowledge and Dr. Deb Zepf's experience in building a business, they developed the following SMART objectives for her complementary alternative business. For Dr. Zepf, the goals and changes led to a significant difference in income, business priorities, self-worth, understanding of the sales aspect of business, and understanding of the value of her services. Dr. Zepf's business changed focus to match her skills and priorities in life. However, the goal of SMART is to develop plans that align with each individual's life and priorities, so they must be created with careful thought for each person.

	Smart Critera	Objectives Types
S	Specific	Build Your Team
M	Measurable	Communication Plan to Team
A	Achievable	Creating Residule Income
R	Relevant	Building Your Business
T	Time Bound	Training Your Team

Being Smart About Business

Let's start out with "smart" goals in planning your business. The SMART goal system is impactful for business planning, project management, and overall growth for yourself as well as your business, because it encourages you to examine your market and evaluate how your business plan stacks up. The acronym SMART stands for:

S – Specific:

- ⚜ The objective must be "specific" – a challenging but attainable improvement over your current level of achievement.
- ⚜ The objective must be stated in quantifiable terms, including timelines and measurements.
- ⚜ Do we consider the objective a challenge but not an "impossible dream"?
- ⚜ Will we have to "stretch" to reach the objective?

M – Measurable:

- ♠ The objective must be measurable so progress can be objectively tracked.
- ♠ What measuring tool will we use? Reports? Data? Figures? Events?
- ♠ Is that measurement tool clear? Concise? Easy to use?
- ♠ Does the tool reduce subjectivity? Will people be able to agree on whether the objective was met?

A – Achievable:

- ♠ The objective must be a stretch over where we are but be realistic. The team must feel confident they can reach the target.
- ♠ Is the objective consistent with our resources and personnel?
- ♠ Does the objective clearly relate to your own guiding principles?
- ♠ Is the objective attainable? If the actions are carried out, will the objective be met?

R – Relevant:

- ♠ The objective must be relevant to other goals and objectives in the company.
- ♠ Does the objective dovetail with the overarching goals of the corporation and your business?
- ♠ Will the objective make a difference and produce meaningful results?

T – Time Bound:

- ♠ The objective must have realistic time frames and be able to be accomplished within a reasonable time.
- ♠ Does the objective contain defined timelines?
- ♠ Do our resources enable us to accomplish the timelines?
- ♠ Can we measure the timelines?

The Soul of Goals

Do you struggle with how to create and or write out a goal? Has year after year gone by and you "beat yourself up" for not accomplishing what you really want to accomplish? Are you stuck on the roller coaster of life and not focusing on what YOU really want?

What is interesting is that most of us take more time in planning a vacation or a party than we do planning our futures! Regardless of what format you follow for creating goals...do something and put it in writing! An old proverb states: "Wishing consumes as much energy as planning." and this statement is relevant to your business plan.

Whatever your financial bracket, current weight, or location in life, defining your goals is intrinsic to making changes. If you are looking at the end of next year, wishing you had created a plan for this year, then stop wishing and start acting! Create a plan that leads to your goals. A simple process to create a plan for successfully achieving this year's goals and ensuring alignment with your spirit and soul are described below. A well-known proverb says: "He who fails to plan, plans to fail," and making solid, aligned goals is the starting point to change.

Planning will occur in one way or another: you will plan, either in the moment (reactive planning) or with a defined plan for your future (proactive). It is always much less stressful to be proactive in planning.

Create a Plan: Use the SMART formula when creating a goal. There are many versions of the SMART Goal formula. Choose what feels right for you!

S - Stands for Specific: This is the what and the how. What are you going to do? Use words such as: create, direct, lead, coordinate, produce, engineer, and organize. How are you going to do it? Use words such as: by, through, and with.

For example: "*I want to make my business profitable.*" "*I want to be successful with essential oils.*" This is too general. Be specific: "*For my business to be profitable, I need to know the exact amount I want to make this year and create a plan that clearly sets weekly monthly and quarterly goals; and take daily steps.*"

M - Stands for Measurable: This is where you will quantify your goal. If you can't measure it, you will not be able to achieve it. Use measures such as: numbers, dates, hours, minutes, and steps.

For example: "*I want to make $50,000 this year, $12,500 per quarter, $962.00 weekly, $137.00 per day working seven days per week.*" This number changes if you only want to work five days per week. Create a plan to hit these numbers. For example, know your profit on every essential oil you sell. Know your overhead because this will subtract from your income. Know your hourly value. How much do you make per massage if you are a massage therapist? Adding essential oils for an additional charge adds value and revenue.

A - Stands for Attainable and Action Oriented:

Peter Drucker states: "Unless commitment is made, there are only promises and hope, but no plans."

There is a balance between stretching and challenging yourself to attain a goal and making it so extreme it becomes impossible to accomplish. Your goals should stretch your comfort zone while still being achievable. **Action Steps** to start working towards this goal need to be listed.

For example (building on the statement above): "I want to make $50,000 in the next twelve months. (see the above financial breakdown) Now let's get more specific (using the counseling profession as an example):

Clarify – financial goals in writing:
- ♠ Know your overhead. What does it cost to run my business? (office space, utilities, internet expenses, essential oils, etc.) Create a spreadsheet.
- ♠ What is my cost for every essential oil? (create a spreadsheet)
- ♠ Am I using essential oils during a therapy session? If yes, what does that cost me, and what will I charge my patient/client? Is it an extra $10 for the session?
- ♠ Am I using a diffuser during the session? What is that costing me?
- ♠ I need to charge X for every counseling session.
- ♠ I need to charge Y for every essential oil I use/sell.

Action – Know the action steps you must take daily:

- ♠ I need to meet with X number of clients/patients weekly.
- ♠ I need to sell X number of essential oils weekly.
- ♠ I need to charge X for the essential oils I use with my patients/clients.
- ♠ I must ensure they take home the blend/essential oils we used during the session.

Calendar – Plan your day. Schedule your success. There is a difference between working <u>IN</u> and working <u>ON</u> the business. Working <u>IN</u> the business is meeting with the clients/patients. Working <u>ON</u> the business is being strategic and action-oriented weekly. Working <u>IN</u> the business is easier than working <u>ON</u> the business.

- ♠ Every business owner must schedule a time to work ON the business weekly. Schedule one to three hours, whatever feels right to you, every Friday to review your week and adjust your plan for the following week.
- ♠ You may need to make phone calls to get more appointments for the

> *"The pessimist complains about the wind; the optimist expects it to change; the realist adjust the sails."*
>
> *– William Arthur Ward*

following week to hit your financial goals.

- ♠ Weekly calendar reviews are necessary to create a successful business.

R Stands for Relevant and Realistic:

- ♠ Is my strategic plan relevant to my personal and or professional purpose?
- ♠ Am I personally and intrinsically motivated to take the needed action to accomplish these goals?

Relevancy is the authenticity check to be sure the goal is in alignment with who you are:

- ♠ Is it harmonious, compatible, and congruent with you and your purpose in life?
- ♠ Is it pertinent to your big-picture goals?
- ♠ Is my strategic financial plan realistic? (*Meaning: is the % of growth/increase, and amount of time to complete a reasonable goal, and do I have the resources?*)

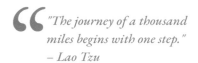

For example (continuing to build on the goal above): "I want to make $50,000 in the next twelve months. I will follow my financial plan stated above; I will schedule time in my calendar weekly to monitor my success and adjust accordingly to hit my goals."
Achieving these goals will:

- ♠ Allow me to serve others on their healing journey
- ♠ Create time and resources for me to accomplish what is important to me and give back to the universe
- ♠ Create financial security
- ♠ Be a philanthropist
- ♠ Align with my core value of encouraging others to seek healing and complete wellbeing

T Stands for Timely: Without a time commitment, we will tend to procrastinate. A clearly defined time frame creates structure and urgency; it gives us a reason to take action now! Having a beginning, an end, and landmarks along the way will keep the momentum going.

For example (completing the statement above): "I will take all the action steps listed above to attain my weekly goal of $_____ and my monthly goal of $_____ and my quarterly goal of $_____ to reach my yearly goal of $_____ by _____(date)."

That is a specific, measurable, attainable, relevant, and timely goal. Sometimes you may have a day or brief time period where you are "derailed" from your goal. *Don't feel defeated. Start again, day by day, step by step.*

The main thing to remember is, what ethics guide your behavior and how do you follow them? Your personal integrity is and will always be the most important code/laws that you have.

Sometimes, you will find it challenging to get started on your goals. Set time aside each day (and week and month) to keep that goal moving forward, even if it is just 15 minutes a week or an hour a month. Those 15 minutes will add up, and slowly you will see real, measurable progress toward your goals.

You will quickly realize if the SMART goal is truly in alignment with your values. If it is not, you will not be motivated, and energy and enthusiasm will dwindle quickly. At that point, you must re-evaluate the goal and go through the process again to find out which piece is not aligned and rewrite the goal (or perhaps let it go). Don't be afraid to say this is the wrong goal or the wrong time for this goal. Goals are good for the soul, so keep your goals in alignment with your inner self and values.

Professionalism in Practice

Professionalism varies these days greatly. From large corporate businesses to single-owner limited liability corporations, many different types of businesses exist, and they hold to different standards of ethics. However, some basics (hopefully) remain the same.

Competence. Ensure your knowledge and experience support your responsibilities–that you have the skills and knowledge to perform effectively.

Reliability. Always show up on time, submit your work according to deadlines, and complete all agreed-upon assignments.

Honesty. Always speak the truth, even when uncomfortable. The more painful ("your product has been delayed and won't arrive for three more weeks") the conversation, the sooner it needs to occur. Be upfront about the entire situation.

Integrity. Be known for your consistent principles.

Respect for others. Treat all people with the same respect, honor, and care as part of your approach, regardless of skin color, sexual orientation, or beliefs.

Self-improvement. Continue to seek education and training in your specialty, and seek to remain ahead of the knowledge curve. New ideas and applications are always evolving; become an interested, lifelong student.

Being positive. Develop and maintain an upbeat attitude, regardless of the pressure. Choosing to be a problem solver makes a big difference.

Supporting others. Share the spotlight with colleagues, take time to show others how to do things properly, and lend an ear when necessary. Give credit to others whenever possible or appropriate.

Staying workfocused. While a personal life is essential, avoid letting your private life negatively impact your job. Avoid using work time to address personal matters.

Listening carefully. Listening to clients and colleagues is important. People want to be heard, so give everyone a chance to explain their ideas adequately.

The Professional Advantage
By encompassing the above points, your reputation as a fair, caring, and ethical practitioner will expand. The additional benefits include increased self-worth and dignity, as well as marketable professional traits.

Knowledge and training are fundamental to success as an aromatherapist. Being prepared, business planning, and personal confidence are also critical assets to win. Every practitioner should stay informed about the aromatherapy world, join associations, attend professional seminars, and read trade journals.

1. **Successful image** is wonderful self-worth and asset. Your personal image should inspire confidence and trust in your client. Appearance, personal grooming, and showing vibrant health and wellbeing are essential to serving others.

2. **First impressions** are also very important. If working out of the home, create a separate, professional space to meet clients. If working from an office, ensure the waiting room is clean and organized, with products displayed for maximum attractiveness and appeal. Ensure good lighting, even if you need to replace fixtures. Consider using a diffuser in your waiting room or office, and note the pros and cons of using one.

3. **Certificates/diplomas** should always be displayed. This gives your prospective new clients and already established clients the assurance of knowledge, background, and completed training from their practitioner. It is not sufficient to say that you are qualified; each client needs to see it.

4. **Develop close, human relationships**. Every person is a spiritual being having a human experience and needs to meet their practitioner at this level.

In addition to being a professionally trained aromatherapist, you must be able to understand a client's needs and build relationships through:

- Good manners
- Pleasant voice
- Cheerfulness
- Tactfulness
- Mindfulness
- Loyalty
- Empathy
- Intuition
- Patience
- Sense of humor
- Assertive
- Maturity
- Interest in the client's welfare
- Confidentiality

We have reviewed the basics of starting a business with a good foundation. A great foundation will last. We are developing our business skills to create an excellent, successful aromatherapy practice, whether exclusively in aromatherapy or adding it as a therapy.

And, there seem to be many different types of professionalism these days! Just look around and notice how many different types of businesses and ethics exist regarding how to run them. Here are some final tips for you:

- **Competence.** You're good at what you do, and you have the skills and knowledge to do your job well.
- **Reliability.** People can depend on you to show up on time, submit your work when it's ready, etc.

- ♠ **Honesty.** You tell the truth and are upfront about where things stand.
- ♠ **Integrity.** You are known for your consistent principles.
- ♠ **Respect for Others.** Treating all people as if they mattered is part of your approach.
- ♠ **Self-Upgrading.** You seek ways to stay current rather than letting your skills or knowledge become outdated.
- ♠ **Being Positive.** No one likes a constant pessimist. Having an upbeat attitude and trying to be a problem-solver makes a big difference.
- ♠ **Supporting Others.** You share the spotlight with colleagues, show others how to do things properly, and lend an ear when necessary.
- ♠ **Staying Work-Focused.** Not letting your private life needlessly impact your job, and not spending time at work attending to personal matters.
- ♠ **Listening Carefully.** People want to be heard, so you give people a chance to explain their ideas adequately.

Having a lot of experience starting small companies, I can tell you that you want to beat the odds and make it a success. A little luck helps, but it does not take away from a good plan and the passion to follow through with it. Those who are running a small business now and want to introduce aromatherapy as a new product and /or service find it a little easier than those starting from scratch.

Adding aromatherapy to an existing company is an excellent business pathway. Our world is constantly changing, and to survive in, our businesses need to evolve and shift product offerings and transaction types, such as offering internet purchases. Many companies refashion into something totally different after 15 years of operation. However, these types of changes need to be made with a business mindset. Keep going back to the business plan and make changes that make sense to meet your soul goals and business priorities.

Chapter 14 References:

Author's Note:
I give much gratitude and thanks to Marguerite Ham that I can bring you this information. Her guidance and insights from "Soul of Goals" and "Smart Objectives" have helped so many on this journey. I hope they help you too. More information on Marguerite is available at: www.MargueriteHam.com

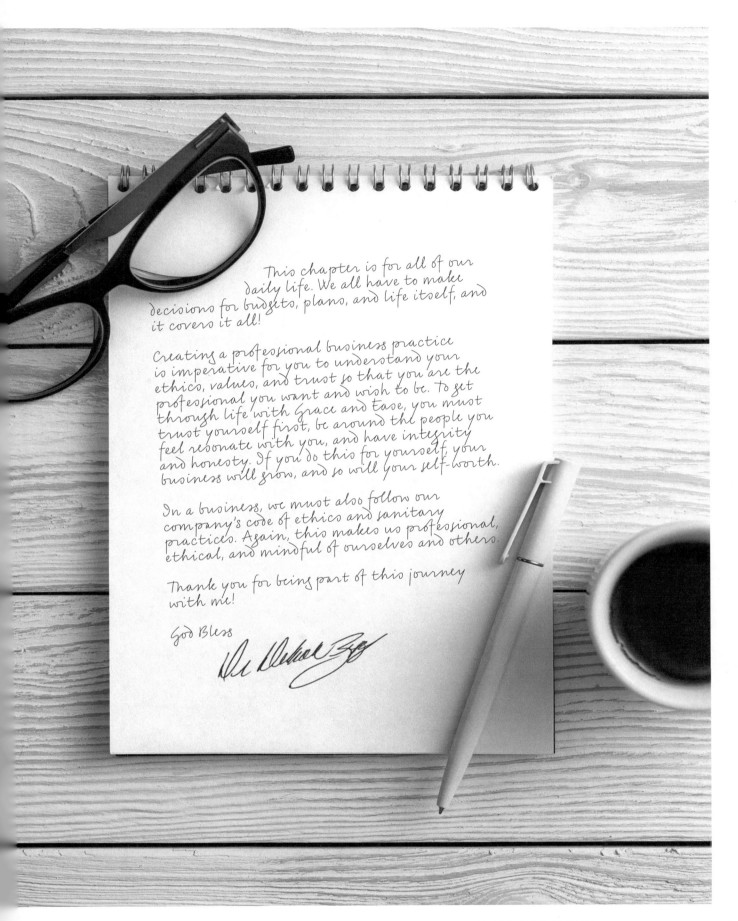

This chapter is for all of our daily life. We all have to make decisions for budgets, plans, and life itself, and it covers it all!

Creating a professional business practice is imperative for you to understand your ethics, values, and trust so that you are the professional you want and wish to be. To get through life with Grace and Ease, you must trust yourself first, be around the people you feel resonate with you, and have integrity and honesty. If you do this for yourself, your business will grow, and so will your self-worth.

In a business, we must also follow our company's code of ethics and sanitary practices. Again, this makes us professional, ethical, and mindful of ourselves and others.

Thank you for being part of this journey with me!

God Bless

INCORPORATING ESSENTIAL OILS INTO YOUR TOOLBOX FOR LIFE

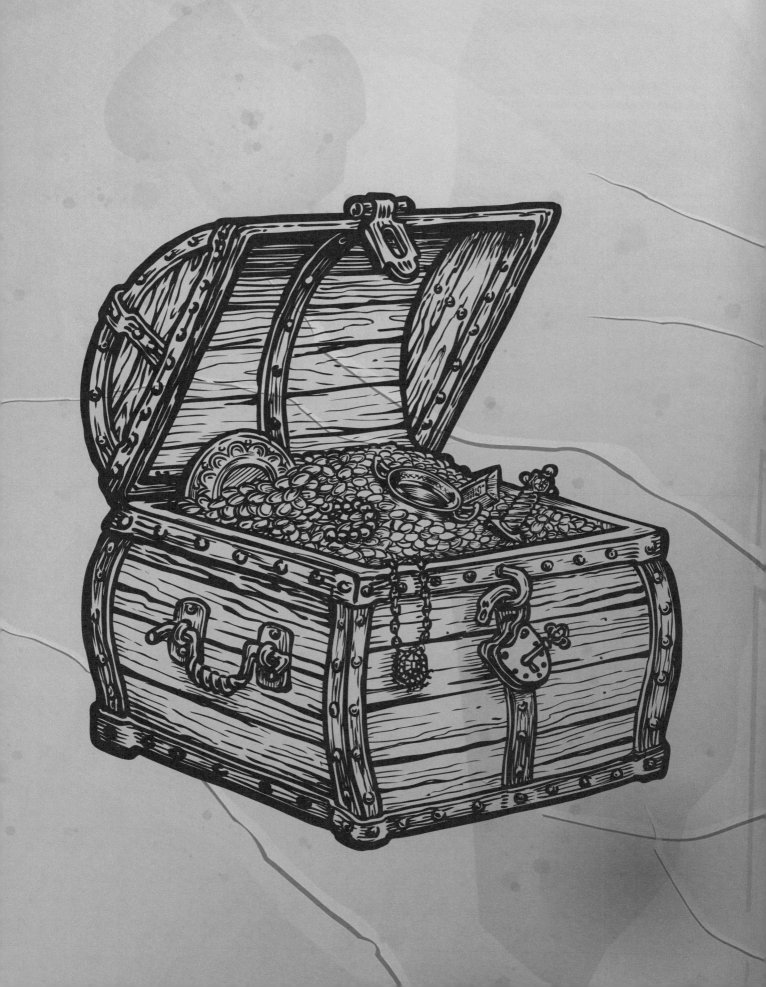

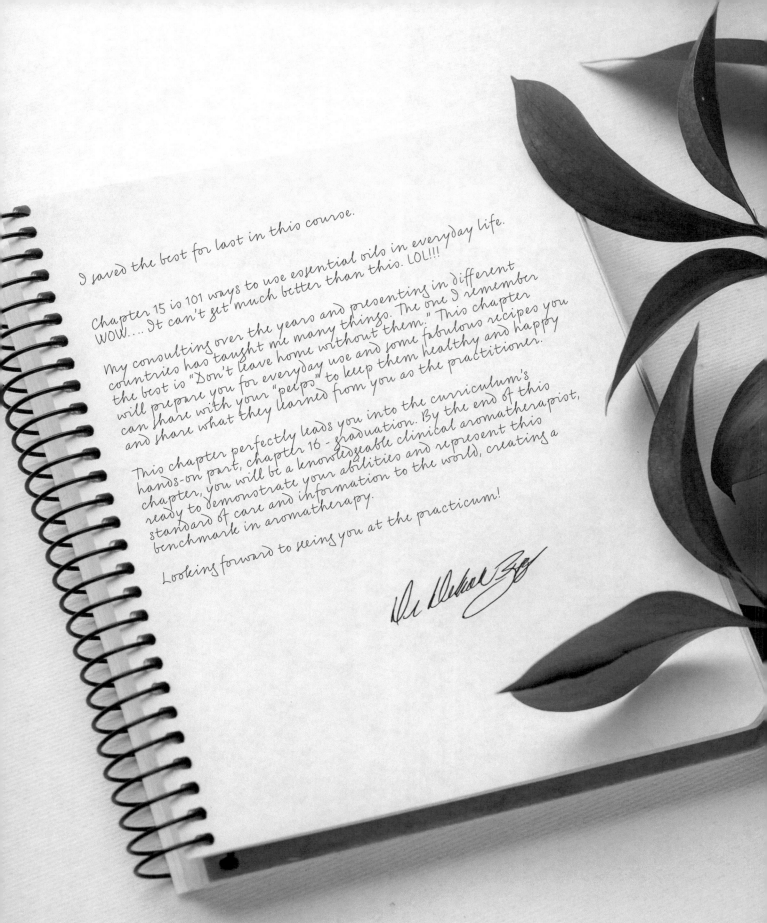

I saved the best for last in this course.

Chapter 15 is 101 ways to use essential oils in everyday life.
WOW..... It can't get much better than this. LOL!!!

My consulting over the years and presenting in different
countries has taught me many things. The one I remember
the best is "Don't leave home without them." This chapter
will prepare you for everyday use and some fabulous recipes you
can share with your "peeps" to keep them healthy and happy
and share what they learned from you as the practitioner.

This chapter perfectly leads you into the curriculum's
hands-on part, chapter 16 - graduation. By the end of this
chapter, you will be a knowledgeable clinical aromatherapist,
ready to demonstrate your abilities and represent this
standard of care and information to the world, creating a
benchmark in aromatherapy.

Looking forward to seeing you at the practicum!

Dr Deborah Bee

CHAPTER FIFTEEN:
INCORPORATING ESSENTIAL OILS INTO YOUR TOOLBOX FOR LIFE

This chapter combines your knowledge, expertise, and experience, coherently and mindfully, into one. As a clinical aromatherapist, you have come a long way to accomplish this goal. You have all of your tools in the toolbox and the pearls of wisdom to achieve anything in life you want and desire as a professional clinical aromatherapist. Whether you are starting a business from scratch, adding it to your present situation, or using them to enhance your and your family's health can be life (and health) changing.

Essential oils can support wellness and health in nearly every area of life. The following suggestions are described for an efficient approach to explaining how to incorporate a healthy lifestyle and a wholesome and nourishing approach to life using aromatic medicine. Moving through the rooms of a house (as well as a few outside activities) shows you how we can incorporate essential oils into every aspect of life for positive, healthy results.

Following the suggestions from this chapter will bring enlightenment and light to your soul to help guide yourself and your loved ones to whole-body positive health.

Encouraging Wellness Throughout Your Home and Life

Whether the residence is a tiny castle off the grid, a house in suburbia, a rural farm, or an apartment in the bustling city, the home is an excellent perspective to describe how essential oils can be incorporated into every area of your life.

One could compare the infrastructure of a house to how the infrastructure of your body (skeleton) supports life. Like calcium strengthens bones, essential oils can provide the baseline support for a healthy environment for living. The following suggestions (and they give only a beginning list) would support the overall health and wellbeing of the residents of a home:

- For a 1,200 to 1,500 sq. ft. living space (scaling up or down according to size), use the following applications for essential oils.
- For each drain in the house, five drops of lemon essential oil with baking soda.
- In the furnace filters, 20 drops of a blend of cinnamon, clove, sweet orange, and peppermint.
- Add a filter in the room vent (assume 12 vents in 1,500 sq. ft.), using five drops of any above blends.

- In the presence of mold, use a 50/50 blend of grapefruit and tea tree essential oils, one tablespoon liquid soap, and a gallon of warm water, and apply the mixture liberally to walls (can be used in a diffuser without the soap).
- To address fungus in bathrooms or bedrooms, wipe the area with a 50/50 blend of sandalwood and a citrus essential oil, such as lemongrass or grapefruit. It can also include sweet marjoram.

Other concerns in the home that can be addressed with essential oils include:

- **Radiation** (*including radon*) - Radiation occurs naturally in the soil and radiation generated from microwaves. As a holistic approach using herbs, cilantro provides amazing support when the body contains heavy metals (i.e., radiation inside the cells). Drink a daily smoothie, adding a large, fresh bunch of cilantro. To address the radiation resulting from cancer treatment/surgery, use the aloe vera plant in association with essential oils. The essential oils are equal amounts (approximately 2 ml each) of helichrysum (Helichrysum italicum) and blue tansy (Tanacetum annuum, annual tansy, not the vulgaris). Create a spritzer and spray the affected area. The large leaf aloe (aloe barbadensis) should be approximately 2 inches wide at the thickest part. Break the leaf at the base and squeeze the "juice" over the spritzed, affected area. If this is to support the body's removal of heavy metals (or radiation inside the cells), the spritz blend should also be applied to pulse points.
- **Electromagnetic Fields** - Electromagnetic radiation is light that travels by oscillating in waves at a constant speed carrying energy, and most electronic devices emit this radiation into the field. There is no scientifically proven evidence to conclude that exposure to low-level electromagnetic fields harms human health. However, international research is currently focused on the possible links between cancer and electromagnetic fields from power lines and radio frequencies. Quantum medicine and natural health professionals have been researching applications to support the body's filtering organs to remove these toxins. Exposure to electromagnetic fields in our homes and everyday lives occurs through:
- **Radio Waves** - used for communication through devices such as television and radio, cell phones, iPads, etc., which are often held close to the head (brain), potentially affecting the central nervous system

- 🍃 **Microwaves** - Microwaves are used for cooking and heating food and satellite communications. Only 90 seconds in a microwave changes the entire molecular structure of the food and compromise the nutrients.
- 🍃 **Visible Light** - Examples of visible light would be incandescent light bulbs, fluorescent lights, and neon lights. While visible light is essential as soon as the sun goes down, we need to understand the effects of artificial light sources on the body.
- 🍃 **Ultraviolet Radiation** - Since this radiation comes from the sun, it is a daily source of exposure and the leading cause of basil cell and squamous cell carcinomas, as well as melanoma. Three UV light rays include UVA (least potent but most abundant), UVB, and UVC (most deadly, but fortunately, most is absorbed by the earth's atmosphere before reaching the surface). For humans, our bodies require the vitamin D produced by exposure to UVB rays to function optimally; however, UVB damages DNA, so limiting exposure is key to healthy skin. Suntans and sunburn are familiar effects of overexposure to the skin, and they ultimately cause wrinkling, leathering, and premature skin aging.

Effective application of essential oil blends to support healing from UV damage would include massage on the feet and over the liver and lung meridian points. Also, hot tea with honey or maple syrup as an emulsifier to distribute the essential oil is a lovely way to embrace healing from the inside out. The essential oils for detox might include the following in a 10 ml blend:

- 🍃 Juniper, three drops
- 🍃 Pine needle, two drops
- 🍃 Bergamot, six drops
- 🍃 Geranium, one drop
- 🍃 Lavender, two drops

Bedroom

The bedroom is significant to overall health and wellbeing. Humans need a minimum of eight hours of sleep daily, and the quality and amount of sleep directly affect the immune system, overall health, weight management due to cortisol/stress, and general mental wellbeing. Essential oils provide support by calming the central nervous systems, allowing the brain to enter deep delta sleep, and effectively allowing the body systems to repair cells at a microcellular during rest cycles. Essential oils also support renewing and regenerating the balances within the cells in the body, restoring cellular communication. Each bedroom should have a diffuser with oils specific to the resident's ages and ailments for effective overnight support.

WARNING: *Overusing these essential oils (8 hours every night) could cause bodily challenges. Ensure that all bedroom occupants are not sensitive to essential oils before use. If there is any oil sensitivity, dilute with a carrier oil or start with half the recommended dosage.*

Children

Children's bedroom over six years of age:

- Lavender, four drops, Roman chamomile, three drops in a diffuser (and four drops of sweet orange and three drops of lavender)

Children 2 to 6 years of age:

- 3 drops of lavender and one drop of myrtle in a diffuser

Children under two years of age:

- only use two drops of lavender on a cotton ball.

Adults

The body heals ONLY while in theta or delta sleep; therefore, choose oils that encourage physical and mental relaxation. An excellent blend for use in a diffuser by the bed at night would be:

- For deep, rejuvenating sleep, use 1:1 lavender and Roman chamomile blend using 10 to 12 drops of the blend in a diffuser with 300 ml of water.
- Also, for use in the bedroom: fractionated coconut oil provides the best lubrication for sexual intimacy—it never goes rancid and provides antibacterial and antiviral properties. Do not include essential oils when using as lubrication.

Elderly over 65

With the elderly, similar precautions should be observed, as noted above, with children with mindful attention to any sensitivity. Check for contraindications to any prescription or over-the-counter medications such as Selective Serotonin Reuptake Inhibitors, which are antidepressants that work by increasing levels of serotonin within the brain.

Bedtime Salt Bowl Method

If the noise from the diffuser is disturbing, or additional moisture in the air is not preferable, the salt bowl method provides an excellent alternative to a diffuser. This method incorporates healing potential into the environment during sleep cycles.

- Place a small amount (about 1/4 cup) of sea salt flakes or Epsom salt in a small bowl.
- Using a pipette or bottle reducer cap, add 10 to 15 drops of your chosen essential oil blend onto the salt.
- Place the bowl by the head of the bed. The salt slows the evaporation rate of the oils, allowing diffusion throughout the night.

Bathroom

Our skin is the body's most significant living organ, and we absorb chemicals and free radicals daily through environmental exposure. The daily time spent in the bathroom brings the opportunity to reverse this damage and build more vital cellular health. Depending on the skin's temperature, the skin absorbs 15 to 25% of the essential oils (Chapter 3). An excellent regimen might include facials (an anti-aging application), warm, relaxing, healing baths, showers, and other skincare.

Facial

For ease of application and clean-up, the facial can be mixed and applied before a bath/shower and then rinsed off after.

- ½ cup of garbanzo bean flour – (chickpea flour)
- ½ teaspoon turmeric
- 2.5% dilution – 15 drops total essential oil/30 ml (1 ounce) fractionated coconut oil
- Lavender, three drops
- Frankincense, one drop
- Geranium, three drops
- Rosemary, two drops
- Myrtle, four drops
- Lime, two drops

The above-mentioned is a blend for normal skin. For sensitive skin, use 1ounce of fractionated coconut oil and 0.5 ounces of avocado oil (facial blend developed by Christie Edwards, Ph.D.)

Mix the flour and turmeric in a container with a tight-fitting lid. Keep in a dry place in or near the bathroom.

To make a mask, combine one tablespoon of the flour/turmeric mixture with five drops of the essential oil blend and five drops of fractionated coconut oil. Add enough water to make the paste similar to the consistency of a cake batter. Apply to the face, using fingers on your face and neck to stay clear of your eyes. Leave on for at least 15 minutes for complete healing properties. However, turmeric can leave orange stains, so be aware of potential skin tinting. Also, wash it off in the shower or bath; it's the best place. Turmeric stains, so please ensure that you are using towels that you won't mind getting stains on.

Goodnight, babyface nighttime moisturizer blend.

After washing off the facial, an overnight moisturizer provides additional care, healing, and anti-aging properties for the skin. Massage gently into the face, neck, and decolletage, and enjoy overnight rejuvenation and repair:

- 2.5% dilution – 15 drops total essential oil blend with 30 ml (1 ounce) fractionated coconut oil or Moroccan oil
- Lavender, three drops
- Frankincense, one drop
- Geranium, three drops
- Rosemary, two drops
- Myrtle, four drops
- Lime, two drops

Bath/Shower (Adults)

Absorbing through respiratory and skin pathways in a warm, soaking bath allows for the highest absorption and most effective healing. Essential oils should be added to the bath water before entering, and the body should be immersed, up to the shoulders, if possible, for at least 15 to 20 minutes to support healthy skin, lungs, and liver.

Using essential oils in the bath creates the maximum absorption for healing for the entire body. The process is two-fold:

Breathing the essential oils incorporates 100% of the healing properties of the oils.

Absorbing essential oils into the body through the skin incorporates 20% of the healing properties.

If you don't have time or the inclination to soak in a warm bath, you can use essential oils with a shower gel, using three drops of a blend on a loofah sponge. The morning (reviving) combination might include sweet orange, rosemary, and lemongrass in a 1:1:1 ratio. A soothing/relaxing blend for nighttime bathing might consist of frankincense, lavender, and sandalwood (1:1:1 ratio). For best absorption, the shower should be warm to hot, and you should breathe deeply for 3 to 5 minutes to ensure maximum absorption and cellular renewal. You can also incorporate the blend into your body wash, using 10 ml per 500 ml of body gel/wash. A morning energizer blend might include sweet orange, lavender, and spearmint (adding 1 ml of this blend into your 16-ounce bottle of body wash)

Basic Bath Recipe:

- 1 cup Epsom salts or sea salt
- Eight drops of Rosemary
- Two drops Lemongrass
- One drop Frankincense
- 1 cup of heavy milk/cream or substitute of milk (i.e., coconut/almond/walnut milk)

Detox Bath Recipes

A bath provides effective double-pathway healing for specific ailments, such as lethargy, skin challenges, insomnia, or other mind and body challenges. Some examples include:

General body detox for lethargy:

- 1 cup Epsom salts
- 1 cup Dead Sea salt
- 1 cup Apple Cider Vinegar
- 1 cup baking soda
- essential oil blend: Juniper (1 drop), Myrtle (4 drops), Lavender (4 drops), Fennel (2 drops)

Hydrogen peroxide bath (skin ailments/softening):

- Two cups of food grade Hydrogen Peroxide
- ½ cup Epsom salts
- 1 cup heavy cream or milk
- essential oil blend: Eucalyptus (3 drops), Frankincense (1 drop), Geranium (1 drop), Pink Grapefruit or Lime (10 drops)

Bentonite clay bath (skin healing and support for eczema):

You can add the bentonite clay and apple cider vinegar directly to the water and site for 10 to 15 minutes. You can also mix apple cider vinegar and bentonite clay to form a paste, then apply it to the skin and soak for 10 to 15 minutes. Either method is messy and will require heavy cleaning after.

- 🍃 1 cup of Bentonite clay
- 🍃 ½ cup Apple Cider Vinegar
- 🍃 essential oil blend: Vetiver (1 drop), Lemon (7 drops), Myrtle (3 drops)

Deodorant

Commercial deodorants/antiperspirants can be effective in preventing sweat stains and body odor, but they often rely on aluminum and formaldehyde, which are detrimental to overall health. Essential oils provide both pleasant scents and reduce overall perspiration without toxicity. An effective application would include fractionated coconut oil (6 drops) with your favorite essential oil (lavender, sweet orange, ylang-ylang, patchouli, or others).

Haircare

For thinning hair, you may add rosemary (1,8 cineol) to shampoo (10 ml per 12 ounces). Do not use it while you are pregnant. Also, applying coconut oil as a mask and leaving for 1 to 2 hours or overnight leaves the hair with a silky feel.

Oil Pulling (Mouth minse)

This application supports gum and tooth health by removing bacteria as well as lymph jaw drainage. One recipe could include one tablespoon of coconut oil or sesame oil, one drop of clove, and two drops of Peppermint. Swish around the mouth for 20 minutes twice daily for 21 days.

Toothpaste

In a 6-ounce container, fill ¾ full of coconut oil. Add three tablespoons of baking soda and 1 ml of your favorite mouth/teeth blend for freshness.

Mouth Rinse/Wash

Combine Neem with electrolytes and, depending on your taste, Peppermint, Spearmint, Wintergreen, Cloves (tooth and mouth pain), and/or Sweet Orange. Add essential oils according to taste, with no more than a 5% dilution.

Body Lotions

Lotions keep our largest living organ healthy and attractive and are especially necessary when living in a dry climate. Dehydration can be determined by the overall dryness of the skin on the hands and feet. To combat dehydration and dryness, drink half your body weight in ounces of water daily and apply lotion all over. Combine Sweet Orange (8 drops) and Cinnamon (4 drops) with 8-ounce unscented Shea Butter for a pleasant-smelling, effective lotion. You can also add one teaspoon of honey, which adds healing properties to the lotion.

Perfume

Most commercial perfumes are made with the scent, not the living, vibrational frequencies that are part of essential oils. They often contain alcohol, aldehydes, and chemicals that can be detrimental to overall wellness. Creating your own perfume enhances your physical, mental, and spiritual wellbeing, and they can be crafted to meet specific system needs. Applying essential oil blends to the pulse points, on your collar bone, on both sides of your neck, and behind your knees sustains scent throughout the day. The blend can also be applied daily to the soles of feet and inside shoes. Your favorite essential oil blend can be mixed in a 20% dilution in a 10-mil roll-on applicator. Blue tansy (1 drop), Pine (2 drops), Sweet Orange (6 drops), Sandalwood (2 drops), and Roman Chamomile (1 drop) are an ancient blend used to bless warriors before leaving for battle. This blend provides grounding and courage for the entire day.

And don't forget to clean your bathroom! Excellent fresh air and deodorizer would be:

- ♠ Lemongrass, six drops
- ♠ Tea Tree; 1 drop
- ♠ Grapefruit, three drops

This blend can be placed in a tablespoon of liquid soap and used to wash walls (mix with 2 gallons of water). Used in a diffuser at full strength, it will help eliminate mold/mildew and viruses/bacteria in the air.

Medicine Cabinet

Preparing with essential oils allows you to treat everyday complaints quickly, safely, and with overall wellness as profoundly as the heart. These aromatic medicines are effective in finding and treating the underlying root cause rather than focusing solely on symptoms of the underlying condition. However, there are also treatments for emergencies, such as minor cuts and bruises. Obviously, for any medical treatment, the practitioner should research any underlying health considerations and review all safety precautions. For children under two years, use only lavender.

Daily aches and pains

Essential oils can provide support and relief for pain caused by inflammation (i.e., the body's reaction to simple cuts and bruises as well as systematic pain caused by arthritis, pancreatitis, cystitis, and other inflammatory-based diseases)

Single note such as Basil ct. linalool (*Ocimum basilicum*) provides analgesic, antispasmodic, balancing, energizing, soothing, and refreshing properties to address muscle spasms, muscle strain, stiff joints, and poor circulation. Basil essential oil should be used in a 20 to 30% dilution.

Single note such as peppermint (*Mentha piperita*) provides analgesic, anti-inflammatory, antispasmodic, and astringent properties to address inflammation. It supports and relieves muscle aches, spasms, sciatica, stiff joints, and menstrual cramps. Blending the two mentioned above with carrier oil may be applied directly to the affected area.

Inflammation blend (in 10 ml carrier oil)
- German chamomile, two drops
- Helichrysum, five drops
- Lavender, two drops
- Peppermint, four drops
- Tea Tree, one drop
- Wintergreen, two drops

The properties of this blend include calming and soothing inflammation and supporting the lymphatic and immune systems.

Joint support and pain relief (in 10 ml carrier oil)

- Eucalyptus globulus, five drops
- Juniper berry, two drops
- Lavender, three drops
- Marjoram, two drops

- ♣ Sweet Orange, Pine, four drops
- ♣ Clove, two drops

This blend warms and soothes joints to promote comfort and mobility.

Massage blend for pain (in 10 ml carrier oil)
- ♣ Eucalyptus globulus, one drop
- ♣ Douglas fir needle, three drops
- ♣ Lavender, two drops
- ♣ Niaouli, five drops
- ♣ Peppermint, one drop
- ♣ Rosemary ct. cineole, one drop
- ♣ Tea Tree, one drop

Muscle soothing and emotional tension blend (in 10 ml carrier oil)
- ♣ Sweet Fennel, two drops
- ♣ Lavender, one drop
- ♣ Lemon, six drops
- ♣ Lemongrass, two drops
- ♣ Peppermint, two drops
- ♣ Rosemary ct. cineole, three drops

The properties of this blend ease muscle tension and promote emotional balance.

Lotions are a great way to support and manage inflammation, chronic pain, bruises, and discoloration.

For arthritis/achy joints and bones, use 30 drops of clove oil, 15 drops of Peppermint, and 15 drops of Citronella in 8 ounces of unscented Shea butter. Under the age of 12, use half of that concentration.

Asthma

Blend two drops of lavender and three drops of frankincense in a tablespoon of olive oil or fractionated coconut oil. Massage on back, chest, and elbows. The diffuser is the most effective support for lung conditions such as asthma, colds, and pneumonia.

Sinus/Cough

Blend the following essential oils (10ml):

- ❧ Thyme linalool, five drops
- ❧ Grapefruit, four drops
- ❧ Tea Tree, two drops
- ❧ Rosemary, three drops
- ❧ Marjoram, two drops

Use these undiluted oils in a steam bowl (or 1 to 2 drops of the blend). Add the blended, diluted oils to a tablespoon of fractionated coconut oil and use it for massage.

Cuts

Put 1 to 2 drops of geranium oil on a small cut to clot blood and stop bleeding. Then apply a bandage.

Once the cut is closed, choose to apply lavender or rose essential oils to support skin regeneration.

Cold/Flu

Neti pots effectively clear sinuses without chemical intervention. Add a pinch of salt to 6 ounces of room temperature distilled or reverse osmosis water with the following:

- ❧ Palmarosa, one drop
- ❧ Rosemary verbenone, one drop
- ❧ 1/4 teaspoon of fractionated coconut oil

To clear chest congestion and support the respiratory system, massage a blend of essential oils into two tablespoons of olive oil or fractionated coconut oil

- ❧ Spanish rosemary, three drops
- ❧ Hyssop, two drops
- ❧ Lemon, six drops
- ❧ Peppermint, two drops
- ❧ Geranium, two drops

For coughs, create homemade cough drops by combining and boiling ½ cup of maple syrup, three tablespoons of glycerin, and ½ cup of honey until it reaches the hard candy stage when dropped in cold water. Remove from heat and drop onto parchment paper using a teaspoon. Add the essential oils as the candy reaches the hard ball stage, just before removing from heat, to ensure the medicinal properties of the essential oils are not damaged by the heat (five drops of lemon, two drops of rosemary [1,8 cineol], two drops of hyssop, and three drops of peppermint)

Fever

Use two drops of essential oil with 1 quart of lukewarm water applied with compresses/sponge bath to bring a fever down. You can also add Manuka honey to calm the spleen. Appropriate cooling oils would include:

- Spearmint
- Lemon
- Lavender
- Tea Tree
- Roman Chamomile

With swollen glands and lymph nodes, use lavender and palmarosa blend (3 drops each) with a quart of warm, distilled or reverse osmosis water and apply using compresses to the throat (or wherever the lymph glands are swollen).

Melancholy and Depression

While medicines to treat these conditions must be prescribed by a physician, essential oils can provide support and healing without the side effects of mainstream antidepressants.

Blend frankincense (3 drops) and black pepper (5 drops) essential oils for use in a diffuser or steam bowl. If adding to a bath, add heavy cream/milk. A few other oils for depression would include clary sage (hormonal), bergamot (brain function), and mandarin orange (uplifting mood). You can use several oils together to keep the blend balanced. Two or more oils are better than one because the phytochemicals in each oil offer different healing properties and allow the body to choose which constituent it needs.

By Occasion

Make a box, or a kit, containing a list of the recommended essential oils for these occasions. Purchase/blend/add these oils when the occasion occurs to avoid deterioration of the essential oils while stored.

Hospital Kit, Emotional and Physical Support

Always be prepared with your toolkit for when emergency medical care is required, particularly if it involves a hospital stay. Having the tools ready and knowing the properties of oils inside your kit will help minimize stress at the hospital and support regular sleep and healing for the patient. The kit should include the following essential oils:

- Mandarin (emotional support, stress release)
- Bergamot (uplifting emotional support)
- Lemon verbena (antiviral/antibacterial)
- Rosemary (lungs and breathing/upper respiratory support)
- Geranium (as an adaptogen, provides uplifting and relief for mental stress; also provides support for bruising)
- Basil (stimulates clarity, helps with sleep, calms the mind, and soothes nerves)
- Sandalwood (provides emotional support and helps with skin regeneration; also purifies spaces.)
- Lavender (sleep and calming)

The oils can be used individually to address specific challenges, but they provide an excellent, general blend as well for a hospital stay. For a short stay, create a blend using four drops of each with 2 ounces of distilled water in a spritzer bottle. The blend for a short stay (1 week) should include approximately 30 drops total. For a longer stay (more than seven days), the 2-ounce sanitizer spray should be more concentrated, using double the amount of oils (approximately 60 drops total).

Pregnancy Kit, Health and Wellness Support

Each expectant mother will have different challenges and specific needs during her pregnancy. An intake survey should include listing all pregnancy symptoms; some mothers experience morning sickness (general nausea) throughout the first trimester, some experience it throughout the pregnancy, and others are never sick. However, symptoms that are common to most pregnancies can safely be supported with essential oils.

Nausea, Massage Oil, and Tea

Nausea often comes with an increase in hormones that support a healthy pregnancy. While perfectly normal, the side effect of nausea can range from simply inconvenient to physically debilitating. Simple support to relieve nausea includes:

- ♠ Sweet orange and grapefruit, one drop each inhaled from a tissue
- ♠ Ginger and Peppermint, one drop each in fractionated coconut oil applied to the feet or big breaths directly from the bottles
- ♠ Lemon and German chamomile, one drop each inhaled from a tissue

Backache, Massage

Along with yoga and specific natal exercise, essential oils will support the movement of the lymphatic system and ease general discomfort. Add lavender and lemon, 15 drops each, to 9 ml carrier oil. Sitting forward over a straight-back chair, a partner and/or friend should gently massage the oil blend into the lower back.

Stretch Marks, Massage Oil

This massage oil blend is wonderfully designed to tonify the uterus, relieve itchiness, and soften skin to minimize stretch marks. Massage a small amount (gently!) in a clockwise direction on the stomach, breasts, and hips. Combine 1 ounce each of sweet almond oil, jojoba oil, cocoa butter, shea butter, and beeswax in an 8-ounce container to make a smooth, silky lotion. Use 1/5 of each base oil/carrier oil to create a 4-ounce bottle. Add the above amounts of essential oils and stir/shake together and voila!

- ♠ Lavender, 30 drops
- ♠ Roman Chamomile, 20 drops
- ♠ Rose otto, ten drops

Birthing Kit, Mental, Physical, and Pain Support during Birth

Aromatherapy can be a wonderful support tool in your toolkit for childbirth. Some essential oils deepen concentration and focus for breathing while also having an analgesic effect. During labor, an anxiety-free atmosphere can facilitate with the help of a diffuser and/or cotton balls around the room with appropriate essential oils such as [1]:

- Neroli encourages easy breathing, calming
- Jasmine for euphoric, antidepressant, uterine healing tonic
- Rose otto as a uterine relaxant (calming to provide more straightforward labor progression), natural antiseptic
- Lavender is a circulatory stimulant, analgesic, calming, antiseptic, anti-inflammatory, promotes wound healing, and relieves headaches.
- Peppermint to support breathing, ease pain and relieve nausea and vomiting
- Clary sage to increase contractions.

Pain Support

Peppermint provides excellent support and can be inhaled by breathing deeply over the bottle or applying one drop of peppermint to the top lip directly under the nose. The oil will support breathing, and the inhalation of peppermint will help ease the pain.

Post-natal Kit, Physical, Mental, and Emotional Support

While larger hospitals may offer a lactation specialist or someone from La Leche League to assist with the baby's first attempts to nurse, continued breast and nipple care at home is essential for the mother's comfort and the wellbeing of the baby. Cracked nipples are a common problem and cause physical (and mental) challenges for both mom and newborn child. Not only are cracked nipples extremely painful, but there is the possibility of infection. This blend of carrier oils can be applied each time after nursing, carefully cleaning off any remaining oil before the next nursing.

- Almond oil, 40 ml
- Calendula-infused oil, 5 ml
- Wheatgerm oil, 5 ml

Near Death/Hospice/Crossing-over Kit

When supporting family or friends anticipating the death of a loved one, this trim kit with perhaps 5 ml of each of the following essential oils can provide comfort and encouragement. These traditional spiritual and worship-related essential oils will help guide and create a safe space for those whose physical bodies are expiring. They will uplift their spirit and soul to a high vibrational frequency, allowing the soul to release from the earth and invite God's presence:

- 🌿 Spikenard
- 🌿 Frankincense
- 🌿 Sandalwood
- 🌿 Atlas cedarwood

Laundry Room

Laundry is a never-ending and rather thankless chore, but it needs to get done, and the more people who live together, the more laundry to get done every week (or every day). Adding essential oils to your laundry regimen helps eliminate odor, mold, mildew, and fungus while keeping the clothes and linens clean and smelling great.

Laundry

In an 8-ounce bottle, blend the following oils and store in the laundry room for easy access:

- 🌿 Grapefruit, 120 ml
- 🌿 Lemon, 100 ml
- 🌿 Tea Tree, 1 ml
- 🌿 Lemongrass, 1 ml
- 🌿 Rosemary, 2.5 ml
- 🌿 Citronella, 2.0 ml
- 🌿 Lavender spika, 0.5 ml (not French lavender, as it is extremely expensive for such a dirty job!)

Add the entire blend to liquid laundry detergent, 8 ounces per 250 ounces of liquid detergent. If using powdered detergent or detergent pods, add 15 drops into each load:

- 🌿 To enhance mental clarity or enjoy the grounding properties and spiritual awareness of your laundry and closet, add five drops of clary sage or frankincense to the laundry blend above

- 🌿 Replace commercially scented softener with plain vinegar

- 🌿 Add five drops of your favorite essential oil per load in the dryer on a cotton ball or dark sock

Living Room

Whether guests or residents of the home, the living room allows interaction, games, movies, and, hopefully, great conversations. Essential oils support and add to a physically, emotionally, and spiritually relaxing ambiance.

Home Diffusers

Essential oils that are used in diffusers throughout the house can add an uplifting, mood-supporting ambiance that touches both the family who lives there as well as guests who enter the home. Add 4 to 15 drops of a sweet orange/grapefruit/lavender blend per day in a diffuser, normally lasting last 6 hours.

Home Office

COVID precautions were a catalyst for changes in the economy and the balance of work performed in centralized offices versus home offices. Essential oils can assist in this new paradigm of working at home, with blends that support focus, creativity, mental acuity, and balance. They can also provide support for stress and anxiety during work pressure and change.

- For mental acuity, use angelica root in a diffuser or 2 to 3 drops on a cotton ball under the desk.
- To combat stress/anxiety and produce overall mental balance, use a blend of helichrysum, sandalwood, and ylang ylang (2 drops each)
- For creativity and focus, use lemon verbena, lemongrass, peppermint, and rosemary, using 1 to 2 drops of each (blend according to preference in scents)

Entryway/Front Door

As an entryway for the world into the home, the mud room/boot room provides a shield or barrier to pollution and contaminants from the environment. It's a great location to store sanitizer in the entryway if a sink is not available for washing hands. It's also the primary location for pet bowls and food, with special consideration for the family's four-legged members.

Pets/Animal Care

Dogs: Special consideration needs to be given when using essential oils on animals. First, they have a much more sensitive sense of smell than humans, and of course, dogs in particular because they come in so many different shapes and sizes. The essential oil blend will differ greatly between a teacup-sized Yorkey versus a Labrador retriever.

Cats: It has become very popular to use aromatherapy with cats. Please be cautious. It's always better to use hydrolats or floral waters. A cat's body weight and size should be considered at all times. Remember that cats are always licking and self-cleaning themselves, so any application of essential oils requires caution.

Leaving Home

Traveling outside the home brings contact with potential contagions and unknown pathogens. Essential oils can support the immune system as well as provide protection from others.

Personal Essential Oil Support

Put a drop of oil on a terracotta pendant, fasten it around your neck, and enjoy the benefits of that oil as you move through your day. You can always use it on your terracotta pots around the house to keep the house fresh and smelling great!

- Blend clove bud, cinnamon leaf, rosemary, lemon, sweet orange, petitgrain, and eucalyptus (1 drop each) and add one drop to mask if using
- Place one drop of lavender on the soles of your feet at the lung meridian point (reflex point to grounding)
- Also, place 1 drop of lemon on the kidney and liver point for uplifting

Environment

Diffusers and cotton balls can be used everywhere with blends for sanitizing, protection, as well as energy and focus while traveling, each with three drops

2-ounce spritzer bottles travel well for airplane use to sanitize seats, tables, and shared surfaces

Unfortunately, bed bugs can be an issue even in nicer hotels and may not be apparent until the bites show up the next day. Spray the bed, carpet, headboard, and other cloth materials in the room. Don't forget the pillowcases and sheets. Once sprayed, leave the room for approximately 1 hour to let the essential oils reach full effectiveness.

- Citronella, 0.5 ml
- Lemongrass, 0.5 ml
- Rosemary (1,8 cineol), 1 ml
- Tea Tree, 0.25 ml
- Thyme (red), 0.25 ml
- Basil linalool, 0.5 ml

- ♠ Bergamot, 1.5 ml
- ♠ Atlas cedarwood, 0.5 ml

Hand Sanitizing Sprays

This sanitizer is not only effective for hands but also safe and effective for toothbrushes, cell phones, door handles, and any area of contact with multiple people, such as grocery carts and automobiles. A 2-ounce spray bottle requires 1 ml of the essential oil blend, using the following sanitizer recipe:

- ♠ Cinnamon leaf, 30 drops
- ♠ Clove bud, 20 drops
- ♠ Ravensara, 40 drops
- ♠ Lemon, 100 drops
- ♠ Tea Tree, ten drops
- ♠ Sweet Orange, 120 drops
- ♠ Black Pepper, 30 drops
- ♠ Oregano, ten drops

Use an 8-ounce bottle to create this blend and have it available to create your 2-ounce spray bottle using distilled water.

Family Travel/Vacations

A travel kit should contain six to eight essential oils that support general challenges encountered during travel. At a minumim it should include:

- ♠ Ginger to relieve nausea.
- ♠ Lemongrass may help to address bug bites and mosquito stings.
- ♠ Rosemary is beautiful for fresh hair and minimizing body odor. It also provides valuable support for mental strain and poor memory.
- ♠ Myrtle may help as an energy balancer to support younger children's respiratory systems.

Also, blend and include the hand sanitizer spritzer for a nightly clean-up before bed.

School
Place a cotton ball or personal diffuser in a lunch box for children (max three drops) with Cypress for focus and mindfulness. Or place one drop on a shirt collar.

Leisure Activities

Essential oils provide support for your environment wherever you travel. Both indoor and outdoor activities provide opportunities for enhancing performance, caring for injuries, and ensuring a positive, uplifting space.

Workouts

Create a spritzer using ten drops of grapefruit, ten drops of lemon, and ten drops of lavender. It will help air out that "exercise room" smell and eliminate bacteria and viruses. Add 4 drops on a tissue and place it in a bag with equipment!

Camping/Hiking

A practical, general kit for camping, hiking, and other outdoor activities should include six to eight essential oils to support common challenges and complaints:

- Lavender provides antibacterial properties, supports cell regeneration, and minimizes discomfort from rashes, blisters, and bruising
- Lemongrass (*citronella nardis*) mixed with geranium and lavender provides excellent bug repellant and relieves itching and swelling from bug bites.
- Lemon, tea tree and citronella ceylon (blended in a 1:1:1 ratio) can be used with a bar of lemon soap to remove the poison ivy oil. Poison ivy surface oil clings to the skin, creating additional irritation if not removed promptly. This blend also relieves other outdoor irritants, including poison oak and bug stings.

Allergies

Outdoor allergies seem to flow and ebb with different seasons and variations in weather. Excellent choices in essential oils to support anti-allergy therapy would include myrtle, which is especially suited for helping red itchy eyes. Unlike most oils/hydrosols, myrtle hydrosol is safe to mist directly on the eyes to relieve itching caused by allergies.

For hay fever, which is another name for allergic rhinitis or a seasonal allergy to pollen/grass, blend these essential oils and apply using a roll-on bottle at a 50% dilution (approximately 3 ml of Neem or fractionated coconut oil):

- Myrtle, cineole type, 2.5 ml
- Hyssop decumbens, 0.75 ml
- German Chamomile, three drops

Apply to wrists, throat, around the ears, and on the chest, legs, and feet for the full anti-allergenic effect.

Kitchen/Dining Room

The kitchen is the heart of the home, especially when the cook is hard at work; family and friends come together to help with the preparation and enjoy conversation and laughter together. Sharing meals, conversation, and laughter in the kitchen create lifelong memories, whether the meals are traditional family favorites or nouveau cuisine. In the kitchen, essential oils can provide nutritional support and enhance culinary taste extravaganzas.

While cooking, use this stimulating, mental creativity blend in a diffuser (2 drops of sage, nine drops of lime, and one drop of Ginger)

To support digestion during the meal, use a diffuser in the dining room area (away from food). Blend three drops of Basil, four drops of Bergamot, and two drops of Black Pepper for the mixture, using 14 to 20 drops in the diffuser

During cleaning the kitchen after dinner, blend one drop of each Clove bud, Rosemary, Lemon, Sweet Orange, Petitgrain, and Eucalyptus. Use 14 drops of this blend in a diffuser in the kitchen.

The kitchen provides a fantastic opportunity for creativity to explore new tastes with essential oils that add flavor and depth to recipes.

Preparing Meals

Breakfast
Smoothies.
Use a maximum of 2 drops for adults (maximum of 1 drop for children 6 to 12 years old), including Peppermint, Citrus oils, and Basil/Thyme, to provide general support for wellness and intense flavors. The oils will also disguise the taste of greens if needed.

Hot Tea.
Add one drop of Ginger and Peppermint to 8 ounces of hot water/tea for digestion support; add to a tea bag, honey, or loose tea leaves rather than directly to the hot water, as you need an emulsifier to distribute the essential oil.

Coffee.
Add essential oils for intense flavors, such as one drop of Peppermint, to coffee grounds or add to creamer or sweetener, such as maple syrup, making a peppermint latte.

Meat Consumption

Adding essential oils to any meat rub you create is a wonderful practice in not only antiviral and antibacterial for your meat, but it creates a wonderful flavor and may support digestion. Adding six drops of black pepper to 1 ounce of ground coffee makes an excellent rub for meat, leaving overnight in the refrigerator for best absorption before cooking. The rub also reduces the toughness of the meat. Black pepper provides support for the mental and emotional aspects of eating.

- Ginger, four drops
- Sweet Orange, 12 drops
- ½ cup of Coco aminos (excellent replacement for soy sauce)
- ½ cup of Sesame oil

This combination creates magic flavors for chicken or stir-fried veggies.

Chicken Balls with maple/orange salsa sauce

- One lb. ground chicken
- 1 tsp basil
- 1 tbsp almond flour
- 1 tsp oregano
- salt and pepper to taste
- One egg
- 1 tbsp ground smoked Hungarian paprika
- 1 cup maple syrup
- 1 cup salsa
- 2 tbsp sesame oil

Essential oils:
- 30 drops of Sweet Orange
- Four drops of Black Pepper

Mix ground chicken with basil, almond flour, egg, oregano, paprika, and salt and pepper. Form into 1-inch balls. Cook at 350° for 30 minutes or until browned—mix maple syrup, salsa, and sesame oil, adding essential oils. Pour mixture over chicken balls and serve hot.

Salad dressing (low calorie and delicious)

- ½ oz of lavender balsamic vinegar
- ½ oz of apple (gravenstein if you can find it), balsamic vinegar
- ½ teaspoon apple cider vinegar
- One oz of lemon olive oil

- ♠ Two drops of Rosemary
- ♠ Two drops of Lemon

Mix well and toss generously with salad before serving. Not only will you have a delicious dressing, but you will also have a healthy one.

Alcoholic Drinks

Kicking Colorado Mule
- ♠ 12oz can ginger beer
- ♠ One oz potato vodka
- ♠ Two slices limes
- ♠ candied ginger

Essential oils:
- ♠ Two drops of ginger
- ♠ Rub the glass with lime and dip in sugar to make a sugar rim. Mix liquids and shake with candied ginger, pour into glass.

Mulled Sangria/Sangria Castaneda
- ♠ Two cups red table wine
- ♠ blackberries for garnish
- ♠ essential oils:
- ♠ One drop of cinnamon bark
- ♠ One drop clove
- ♠ One drop lemon
- ♠ Heat wine, then add oils. Serve with blackberries for garnish

Sage Mojito
- ♠ One oz rum
- ♠ 12 oz club soda – lime flavor
- ♠ Two tsp maple syrup
- ♠ + fresh lime for garnish

Essential oils:
- ♠ One drop Peppermint
- ♠ Two drops Lemon
- ♠ One drop Lime
- ♠ One drop Sage
- ♠ Mix, and serve with a lime garnish

Very Bubbly
- 10 oz blackberry champagne
- small container of blackberries

Essential oils:
- One drop Lavender
- Two drops Lemon

Cook blackberries with 1 tsp lemon juice until fully muddled. Add one tablespoon per champagne glass and serve.

Grateful Lemon Drop Martini
- 1/2 oz Grand Marnier
- 1/2 cup vodka
- 2 tbsp maple syrup
- Juice from half a fresh lemon

Essential oil:
- Two drops of basil
- Mix and serve over ice with basil garnish.

Goodnight Kiss
- 1 oz Kahlua
- 1 oz hazelnut liquor
- 3 oz coconut milk

Essential oil:
- Two drops of Black Pepper
- Mix and serve over ice

Nutty Orange Side Car
- 1/2 oz hazelnut schnapps
- 3 oz coconut milk
- Splash of lime soda
- Orange for garnish

Essential oil:
- One drop of Sweet Orange
- Mix and serve over ice with an orange garnish.

Citrus Tequila
- 1/2 oz triple sec
- 1 oz tequila
- 2 oz soda water with lime flavor

Essential oils:
- ♠ One drop lime
- ♠ One drop lemon

Mix all the ingredients and the essential oils. Use lime to wet the glass rim, dip in salt flakes, and then pour citrus tequila into the glass.

Additional Toolkit Uses

Along with these uses for essential oil in the homes, numerous opportunities are present in our community, cities, and businesses to support others' quality of life and wellness:

- ♠ Funeral homes
- ♠ Hospitals
- ♠ Health clinics
- ♠ Hospice environment
- ♠ Train stations
- ♠ Bus stations
- ♠ Shopping centers
- ♠ Churches/temples
- ♠ Workout/gym facilities
- ♠ Spas

Regardless of the location, the following considerations should always affect the choice of specific essential oils for safe use. The essential oils should be carefully chosen to meet personal/environmental challenges without potential harm to individuals based on the following conditions:

- ♠ Air toxicity
- ♠ Eye health
- ♠ Sinus/mold
- ♠ Lungs
- ♠ Brain
- ♠ Liver
- ♠ Kidney
- ♠ Skin
- ♠ Emotional
- ♠ Spiritual
- ♠ Mental
- ♠ Male and female hormone balancing
- ♠ Ages of all children and elderly (safety precautions)

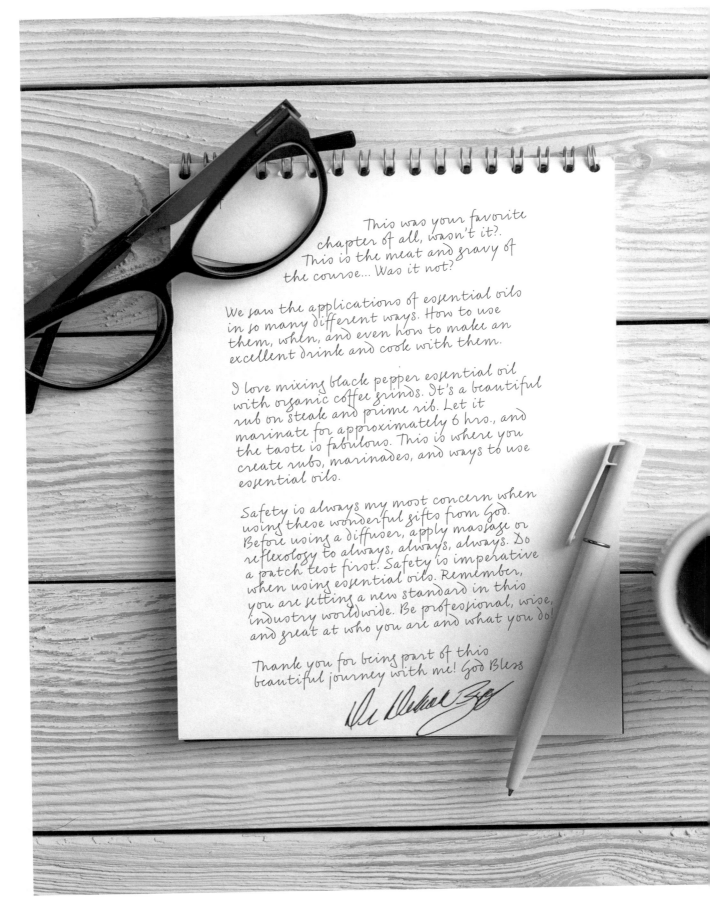

This was your favorite chapter of all, wasn't it?. This is the meat and gravy of the course... Was it not?

We saw the applications of essential oils in so many different ways. How to use them, when, and even how to make an excellent drink and cook with them.

I love mixing black pepper essential oil with organic coffee grinds. It's a beautiful rub on steak and prime rib. Let it marinate for approximately 6 hrs., and the taste is fabulous. This is where you create rubs, marinades, and ways to use essential oils.

Safety is always my most concern when using these wonderful gifts from God. Before using a diffuser, apply massage or reflexology to always, always, always. Do a patch test first! Safety is imperative when using essential oils. Remember, you are setting a new standard in this industry worldwide. Be professional, wise, and great at who you are and what you do!

Thank you for being part of this beautiful journey with me! God Bless

Dr. Deborah Biggs

Chapter Fifteen References:

[1] Battaglia, S., *The Complete Guide to Aromatherapy*, Perfect Potion Publisher, page 447.

Authors Note: (*Burns and Blamey evaluated the benefits of essential oils in a labor ward during their research and the essential oils used included.*)

ESSENTIAL OILS AND THEIR CONSTITUENTS: PART TWO

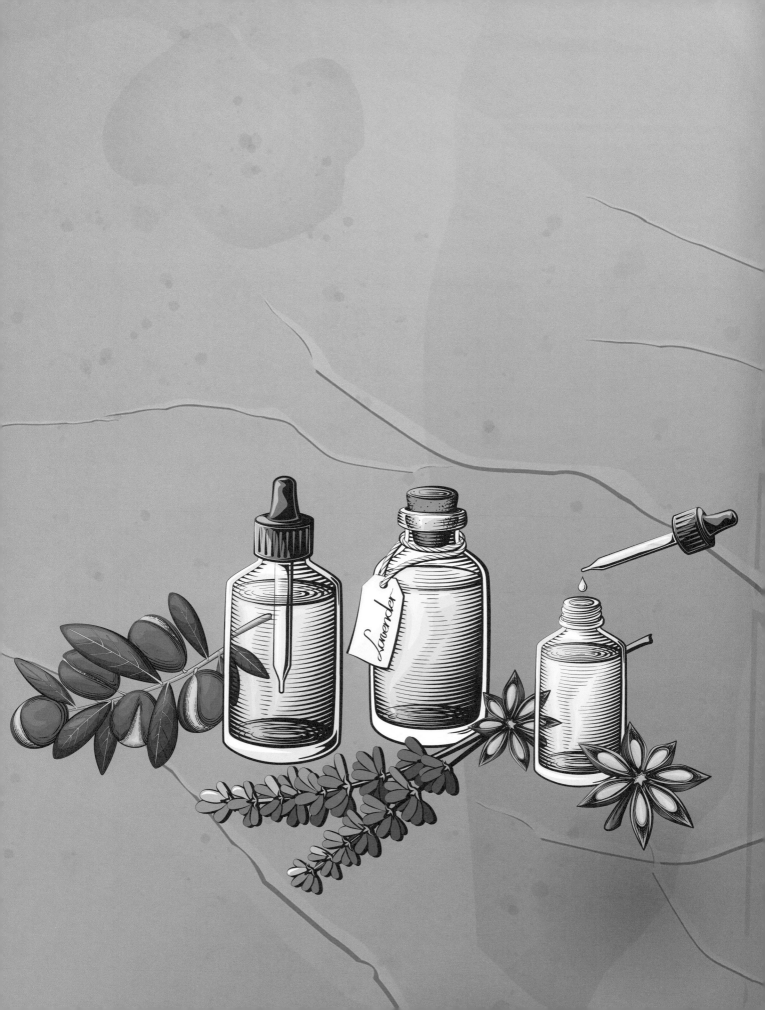

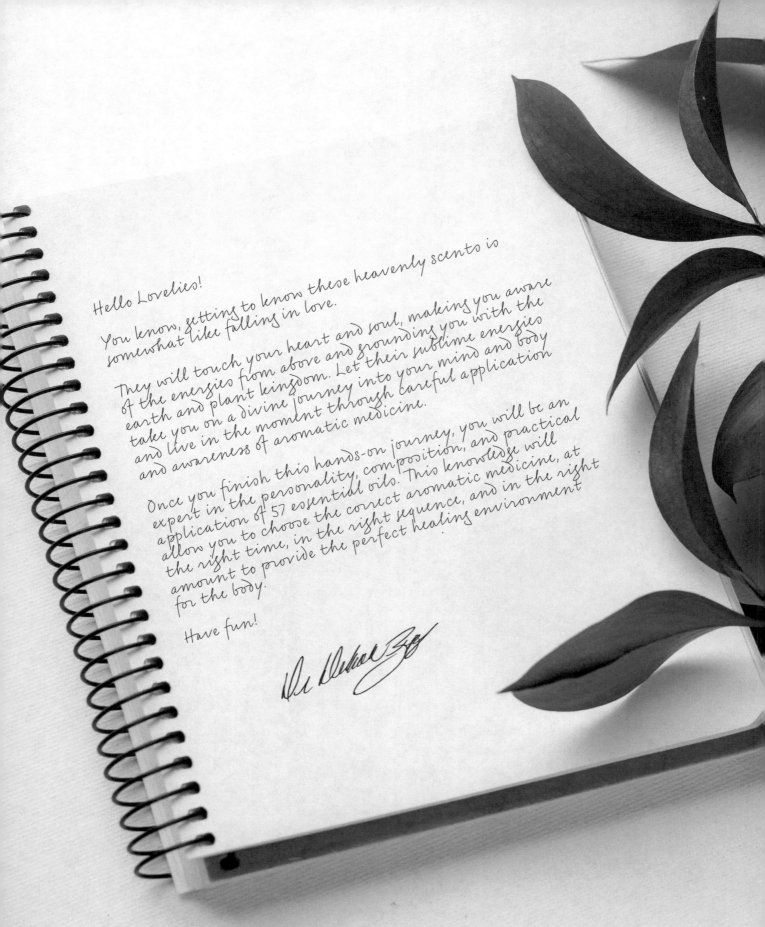

Hello Lovelies!

You know, getting to know these heavenly scents is somewhat like falling in love.

They will touch your heart and soul, making you aware of the energies from above and grounding you with the earth and plant kingdom. Let their sublime energies take you on a divine journey into your mind and body and live in the moment through careful application and awareness of aromatic medicine.

Once you finish this hands-on journey, you will be an expert in the personality, composition, and practical application of 57 essential oils. This knowledge will allow you to choose the correct aromatic medicine, at the right time, in the right sequence, and in the right amount to provide the perfect healing environment for the body.

Have fun!

Dr. Deborah Berg

CHAPTER SIXTEEN:
ESSENTIAL OILS AND THEIR CONSTITUENTS: PART TWO

Welcome to the final step of becoming a Certified Professional Clinical Aromatherapy Practitioner! I hope that you have found this journey exciting and arduous, discovering the tenacity to fully understand essential oils chemical composition and healing potential while embracing the marvelous journey of plant fragrances.

God created all things on this planet, and we heal using the natural vibrational frequencies of the creation. Embrace the natural essence and healing frequencies of these essential oils to raise your own physical, mental, and spiritual vibration to a higher frequency and guide others to wellness.

"Aromatherapy has the basis of the plant and the constituent molecules which possess a chemical intelligence that speaks directly to the human organism" [1].

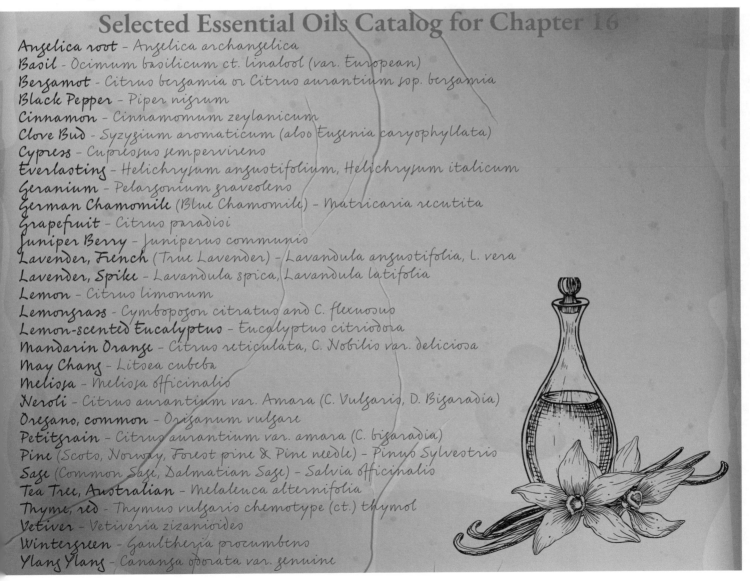

Selected Essential Oils Catalog for Chapter 16

Angelica root - Angelica archangelica
Basil - Ocimum basilicum ct. linalool (var. European)
Bergamot - Citrus bergamia or Citrus aurantium sop. bergamia
Black Pepper - Piper nigrum
Cinnamon - Cinnamomum zeylanicum
Clove Bud - Syzygium aromaticum (also Eugenia caryophyllata)
Cypress - Cupressus sempervirens
Everlasting - Helichrysum angustifolium, Helichrysum italicum
Geranium - Pelargonium graveolens
German Chamomile (Blue Chamomile) - Matricaria recutita
Grapefruit - Citrus paradisi
Juniper Berry - Juniperus communis
Lavender, French (True Lavender) - Lavandula angustifolia, L. vera
Lavender, Spike - Lavandula spica, Lavandula latifolia
Lemon - Citrus limonum
Lemongrass - Cymbopogon citratus and C. flexuosus
Lemon-scented Eucalyptus - Eucalyptus citriodora
Mandarin Orange - Citrus reticulata, C. Nobilis var. deliciosa
May Chang - Litsea cubeba
Melissa - Melissa officinalis
Neroli - Citrus aurantium var. Amara (C. Vulgaris, D. Bigaradia)
Oregano, common - Origanum vulgare
Petitgrain - Citrus aurantium var. amara (C. bigaradia)
Pine (Scots, Norway, Forest pine & Pine needle) - Pinus Sylvestris
Sage (Common Sage, Dalmatian Sage) - Salvia officinalis
Tea Tree, Australian - Melaleuca alternifolia
Thyme, red - Thymus vulgaris chemotype (ct.) thymol
Vetiver - Vetiveria zizanioides
Wintergreen - Gaultheria procumbens
Ylang Ylang - Cananga odorata var. genuine

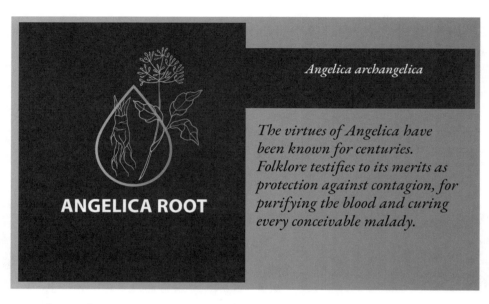

Angelica archangelica

The virtues of Angelica have been known for centuries. Folklore testifies to its merits as protection against contagion, for purifying the blood and curing every conceivable malady.

Angelica Root
Angelica archangelica

It was held a sovereign remedy for poisons and all infections and maladies. Angelica was closely linked with followers of the Christian faith. According to one legend, angelica was revealed in a dream by an angel to cure the plague. Another explanation for the name of this plant is that it bloomed on the day of Michael the Archangel and was used in-house as protection against evil spirits and witchcraft. The powdered root is extensively used in herbal preparations to treat bronchitis, pleurisy, and other diseases of the lungs. It is also recommended for menstrual regulation. [2]

Angelica root is a stout biennial or perennial herb that grows up to 2 meters tall with a large rhizome. According to Battaglia, it is cultivated in Belgium, Holland, France, Germany, Hungary, and northern India. It is preferable that the oil be distilled from roots that are not more than two years old; the quality of the oil changes the age of the root. The oil from older roots provides a different scent, typically sweeter than that from younger roots, but the oil itself is not inferior and provides the same healing properties. [2]

Growing up to 6.5 feet in height, the angelica plant is an impressive sight that bursts with power and energy. The main stem can grow up to 7 inches in diameter with leaves that spread expansively from the stem. The strong root system is deeply anchored in the earth, and the oil brings vital grounding elements. Its crowning glory is a greenish-white, umbelliferous flower. The plant's strong aroma creates a distinctive, easily identified scent. [3]

According to Fischer-Rizzi, angelica was a favorite medicinal plant in the Middle Ages, and physicians used the oil to protect themselves from infections. According to Paracelsus, angelica essential oil was used as a prophylaxis for those who cared for the afflicted during the bubonic plague. To guard against viruses, take 1 to 2 drops of essential oil during the flu season, or use the essential oil in an aroma lamp in combination with lemon or eucalyptus oil when many people gather in a room. [4]

1. **Class:** Monoterpenes

2. **Family:** *Umbelliferae* or *Apiaceae*. Comprising 434 genera and about 3,700 species, the *Apiaceae* family is a significant group of flowering plants. Its members are often aromatic and are characterized by hollow stems, taproots, and flat-topped flower clusters known as umbels. The family of mostly aromatic flowering plants is named after the type of genus Apium and commonly known as the celery, carrot or parsley family, or simply as umbellifers.

3. **Distillation/Method of extraction:** Angelica root oil is steam distilled from the dried roots of *A. archangelica*

4. **Biochemicals:**
   a. Monoterpenes (approx. 70%) α- & β-pinenes (24 &>1.5%) Limonene.
   b. Esters (up to 2%) bornyl and trans-verbenol acetate: terpenoid alkaloids: nitro-menthadenes
   c. Furocoumarins: (about 2%): umbelliferone, archangelicine, angelicin, bergapten, osthol

5. **Uses:** No traditional uses of this essential oil are documented. Most of these are for whole herbal extract uses.
   a. Antiseptic
   b. Antispasmodic

c.   Aphrodisiac
d.   Anticoagulant
e.   Bactericidal
f.   Carminative
g.   Cholagogue
h.   Depurative,
i.   Diaphoretic
j.   Digestive
k.   Diuretic (herbal)
l.   Emmenagogue
m.   Expectorant
n.   Febrifuge
o.   Hepatic
p.   Nervine
q.   Sedative (local CNS support for abdominal spasms)
r.   Stomachic
s.   Tonic: stimulant (digestive)

6. **Chemical composition:** Angelica root chemistry is quite complex. The oil contains up to 70% monoterpenes, hydrocarbons, small quantities of esters, alcohols as well as coumarins and lactones. The furocoumarins found in angelica oil are umbelliferon, archangelicine, angelicin, and bergaptene. These constituents are responsible for angelica's phototoxicity. Coumarins have a strong affinity with the nervous system and can raise the threshold from which one registers nervous stress. [5] The typical chemical composition of angelica root is reported as follows:

a.	α-pinene	21.12 – 25.24%
b.	camphene	1.42 – 1.43%
c.	sabinene, 8-3-carene	7.94 – 10.38%
d.	α-phellandrene	2.38 – 9.58%
e.	myrcene	4.00 – 4.62%
f.	limonene	8.54 – 11.53%
g.	β-phellandrene	14.04 – 16.03%
h.	cis-ocimene	0.24 – 0.38%

i.	trans-ocimene	0.9 – 2.12%
j.	paracymene	6.25 – 11.3%
k.	terpinolene	0.28 – 0.38%
l.	copaene	0.93 – 1.29%
m.	bornyl cryptone	0.44 – 0.99%
n.	α-bisabolene	0.09 – 0.19%
o.	rho-cymen-8-ol	0.14 – 0.35%
p.	humulene monoxide	0.28 – 0.21%
q.	tridecanolide	0.58 – 0.81%
r.	pentadecanolide	0.87%

7. **Systems:**

   a. Integumentary: (skin, hair, nails): Provides support for dull irritated inflamed congested skin, psoriasis, fungal infections, general skin tonic. According to Battaglia, angelica root essential oil is not commonly used in skin care. However, the oil is used as a fragrance ingredient in soaps, detergents, creams, lotions and perfumes. [6]

   b. Respiratory: Provides support for chronic bronchitis, pleurisy, coughs, nervous asthma, shortness of breath, smoker's cough, restores sense of smell, general lunch tonic.

   c. Muscular/skeletal: Supports and relieves symptoms of arthritis, sciatica, and rheumatism.

   d. Cardiovascular/lymphatic: Serves as a circulatory stimulant, blood thinner (works especially well to help remove heavy metals and accumulations of toxins including uric acid), aids white blood cell formation, and warms the body.

   e. Immune: Provides excellent support for colds, fever and flu. Stimulates the lymphatic system, especially to detoxify after illness. Works well with contagious diseases such as typhus, malaria, diphtheria, cholera, and yellow fever. According to Battaglia, angelica root oil is reputed to have excellent detoxifying and diuretic properties. Used in massage oil to improve lymph drainage; relieves rheumatism and arthritis, fluid retention, and cellulite. [7]

f. Digestive: Provides support for anemia, anorexia, (stimulates the appetite), flatulence, indigestion and nausea and bloating discomfort ulcers, colic, and serves as a general tonic for the liver and spleen. Control uric acid: it seems to favor pepsins and hydrochloric acid production.

g. Endocrine: Adrenal sedative

h. Genito-urinary/reproductive: Works well with edema, simple water retention, gout, urinary antiseptic, (cystitis), encourages estrogen for regulating menstruation, painful periods, and may help to expel after-birth. May be useful for infertility in male and female and may help to control uric acid.

i. Central nervous system: Works well with fatigue, exhaustion, migraine, anxiety, and nervous tension. Provides support for fatigue, insomnia, stress-related disorders. Can be used as a pain reliever for headache and toothaches. Promotes a feeling of balance, supports relief from heartache. Can also provide support for recovering alcoholics dealing with cravings for alcohol. [8]

8. **Personality:** According to Fischer-Rizzi, Angelica root will assist people who are afraid, weak or who lack perseverance and have a tough time making decisions. "Don't give up! Stick with it! Don't be afraid – begin to rebuild. You are strong and nothing will knock you down!" The source of angelica's strength is the earth, since the plant itself has been strongly influenced by the elements of the soil. As an essential oil, angelica has a fiery temperament and lends us more physical vitality or earthly strength than cosmic or spiritual energy. Angelica is particularly suited to people who need solid grounding and who search for reality. [9]

9. **Safety:** Photo toxic and possible irritation to skin. Avoid use with diabetes and/or pregnancy. Overuse causes insomnia. Caution: possible irritant and skin sensitizer.

10. **Blending:** Base note.

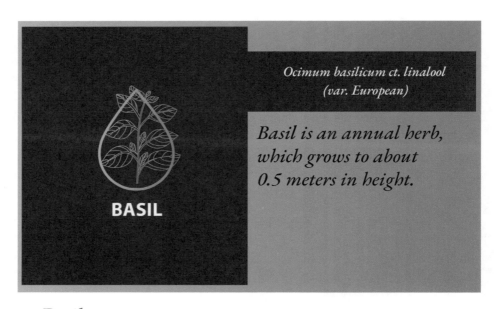

Ocimum basilicum ct. linalool (var. European)

Basil is an annual herb, which grows to about 0.5 meters in height.

BASIL

Basil
Ocimum basilicum ct. linalool (var. European)

It is a native to tropical Asia and Africa. Many varieties of basil are cultivated around the world in multiple climates. Each variety produces a unique essential oil, and the characteristics are determined by environmental factors such as temperature, geographic location, soil, and the amount of rainfall/irrigation.

According to Leung, the two most common basil essential oils found in aromatherapy are[10]:

- True sweet basil oil (European). This oil has a higher percentage of linalool. This oil is generally regard as safe to use in aromatherapy.
- Exotic or reunion basil which is distilled in the Comoro islands Malagasy republic, Thailand and occasionally in the Seychelles. This oil has a higher percentage of methyl chavicol and should be used with caution

Basil essential oils are produced from several varieties and species, and they can exhibit differing properties. Always request GCMS sheets from essential oil suppliers to confirm the correct biochemical constituents and the full range of properties for each essential oil based on the type of plant harvested. The information provided in the chart below for each of the seven basil types will allow the practitioner to select the appropriate, effective remedy for physical and mental challenges from the seven different types listed. The expanded information provided for this classification defines characteristics for all seven varieties of basil essential oils, and the linalool type.

Variety/Origin	Active molecules	Properties	Indications
Ocimum basilicum var. basilicum – (exotic type) Comoro Island Vietnam	methyl chavicol, linalool, eugenol	antispasmodic, active on sympathetic nervous system, anti-inflammative, antiviral	gastritis, pancreatic insufficiency, viral hepatitis types a & b, travel sickness, prostatitis, urinary tract infections
Ocimum basilicum var. grand vert – France	methyl chavicol, methyl eugenol, β-caryophyllene	strongly antispasmodic	colitis, spasmophilia
Ocimum basilicum var. minimum – India	methyl chavicol, methyl eugenol, β-caryophyllene, neral alpha & β-pinenes, citronellal, geranial	antispasmodic, anti-infectious	spasmodic colitis
Ocimum gratissimum (eugenol type) – East India	cis- & trans-β-ocimenes, β-caryophyllene, alpha & β-santalene, eugenol, methyl chavicol	anti-infectious, bactericidal, viricidal, parasiticidal, neurotronic, hormone-like	enterocolitis, intestinal parasitosis, hepatopancreatic insufficiency, prostate congestion, arthrosis
Ocimum gratissimum (thymol type) – West Africa	paracymene, α-thujene, myrcene	general stimulant, strongly anti infectious	cystitis, bronchitis, enterocolitis
Ocimum basilicum var. European/ basilicum (linalool type) – France	cis-3-hexinol, linalool, fenchol, eugenol, methyl chavicol, 1,8 cineol	tonifying, carminative, hepato-stimulant, neurotonic	coronary weakness, nervous depression, liver, gall insufficiency
Ocimum sanctum – Holy basil (sacred basil) – India	eugenol, methyl eugenol, β caryophyllene, β elemene	antibacterial, anti-infectious, antiseptic, antispasmodic calmative, carminative, pectoral, restorative	muscular spasm and contraction, respiratory conditions, cystitis, intestinal spasm, parasitic infection, cramps, menstrual cramps, menstrual problems, headache, migraines, mental and physical fatigue

(Schnaubelt[11] and Worwood [12])

1. **Class**: Alcohol, phenols ethers

2. **Family**: *Labiatae* or *Lamiaceae*

3. **Distillation**: Basil oil is steam distilled from leaves and flowering tops.

4. **Biochemicals**:
    a. Monoterpenes: (2%) α- & β-caryophyllene
    b. Sesquiterpenes: iso-caryophyllene, β-caryophyllene, β-elemene
    c. Alcohols: (up to 65%) cis-3-hexenol, linalool (>55%) fenchol (<10%)
    d. Esters: (<7%): linalyl, fenchyl acetates: methyl cinnamate
    e. Phenols: (6%) eugenol
    f. Phenol methyl-ethers: (<15%) methyl chavicol (up to 47%), methyl eugenol
    g. Oxides: (6%): 1,8 cineol

5. **Uses**:
    a. Analgesic
    b. Antidepressant
    c. Anti-infectious
    d. Antiseptic
    e. Antispasmodic
    f. Carminative
    g. Cephalic
    h. Digestive
    i. Decongestant (prostate and uterus)
    j. Emmenagogue
    k. Expectorant
    l. Febrifuge
    m. Galactagogue
    n. Nervine
    o. Prophylactic
    p. Restorative
    q. Stomatic
    r. Sudorific
    s. Tonic: general

6. **Chemical Composition:**
Estragole is also known as methyl chavicol, and this chemical presents safety concerns as a potential carcinogen as well as presenting contraindications during pregnancy. Therefore, when treating body challenges, the linalool chemotype is a safer choice. The phenolic ethers found in basil provide antispasmodic properties, which are ideal for treating spasmodic abdominal pain and asthmatic conditions. The typical chemical composition of three of the linalool basil oils are:

Compound	Origin		
	Comoro Island	France	Egypt
α-pinene	0.18%	0.11%	0.25%
camphene	0.06%	0.02%	0.07%
β-pinene	0.25%	0.07%	0.43%
myrcene	0.12%	0.13%	0.35%
limonene	2.64%	2.04%	4.73%
cis-ocimene	2.52%	0.03%	0.63%
camphor	0.37%	1.43%	0.57%
linalool	1.16%	40.72%	45.55%
methyl chamicol	85.76%	23.79%	26.56%
α-terpineol	0.84%	1.90%	1.09%
citronellol	0.65%	3.57%	1.76%
geraniol	0.03%	0.38%	0.20%
methyl cinnamate	0.05%	0.34%	0.25%
eugenol	0.74%	5.90%	5.90%

(Battaglia [13])

7. **Systems:**
    a. Integumentary (skin, hair, nails): Serves as an insect repellant. Supports hair growth. Provides renewal and support for a sluggish complexion, dry skin, acne, and eczema. May also provide relief for herpes and shingles infections. Acts as a general skin tonic and provides relief from insect bites.
    b. Respiratory: Provides support for whooping cough, sinus congestion (restores sense of smell with catarrh), asthma, bronchitis, general coughing symptoms, and earaches.
    c. Muscular/skeletal: Provides support for muscular aches and pains including deep muscle spasms. May help with rheumatoid arthritis and rheumatism.
    d. Cardiovascular: Stimulates blood flow, works as a heart tonic, and serves as a decongestant for veins and pulmonary arteries. May be helpful with hypotension, varicose veins, tachycardia, and atherosclerosis.
    e. Immune: Provides excellent support for colds, fever, flu infections.
    f. Digestive: Provides support and relief from vomiting, gastric spasm, hiccups, gastritis, and ulcers. It supports cleaning the intestines, easing migraines resulting from liver and gallbladder challenges, and providers support for gout while stimulating the pancreatic enzymes to lower acidity.
    g. Endocrine: Provides support to regulate adrenal cortex (works as a stimulant.)
    h. Genito-urinary/reproductive: Provides support for cleaning kidneys and aid in cystitis. Eases uterine (and prostate) congestion, cramps, and scanty periods. Also relieves breast engorgement.
    i. Central nervous system: Provides support for anxiety, hysteria, nervous depression, asthenia,

fatigue, insomnia due to nervous tension. It acts as a wonderful tonic and aids clarity of thought, strength of memory and eases "cold" feelings (e.g., feelings of separation and loneliness).

8. **Personality**: Whether male or female, basil personalities are often entrepreneurs of the world and able to see opportunities that others don't even know exist. Ambition, charisma, personal drive, and enterprise will move these individuals forward in life to meet their goals. Unless someone interferes with their work/life unjustly, these individuals will reach life goals without harming others and will be honest in their endeavors. Their character is uplifting, awakening, clarifying and stimulating. This oil supports the attributes of positivity, purposefulness, concentration, assertiveness, and it can be used to counteract negative attributes including indecision, mental fatigue, mental exhaustion, negativity, lack of direction, fear, burnout confusion, intellectual fatigue, bitterness, resentment, fear of intimacy, shame, doubts [14].

9. **Safety**: Avoid using basil during pregnancy. Avoid using basil with high contents of methyl chavicol and methyl cinnamate as it will be an irritant to people with sensitive skin.

10. **Blending**: Top note.

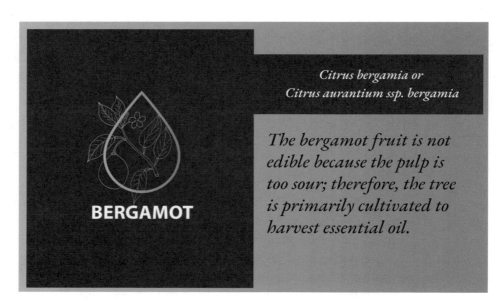

Citrus bergamia or Citrus aurantium ssp. bergamia

The bergamot fruit is not edible because the pulp is too sour; therefore, the tree is primarily cultivated to harvest essential oil.

Bergamot
Citrus bergamia or Citrus aurantium ssp. bergamia

Bergamot is a wonderful perennial flower and plant. The origins of the word "bergamot" are shrouded in mystery. Some researchers suggest the name was derived from the shape of a fruit that resembles the bergamot pear. Others suggest that Christopher Columbus brought it from the Canary Islands to the city of Berga, in the province of Barcelona, Spain and it was introduced from there to Calabria in southern Italy, the principal growing region. But where would Columbus have harvested the bergamot to bring to Spain? Another source suggests the tree is named after the city of Bergamo in northern Italy where the oils was first sold. Wherever the origin, this beautiful plant has been used in Italian folk medicine for the treatment of fever and worms [15]. Approximately 90 percent of the world's crop is produced in the Reggio di Calabria region of Italy, or on the nearby island of Sicily.

The tree cannot be propagated by seed; rather, bergamot buds are grafted onto other citrus rootstocks (normally bitter orange). Some growers believe that lemon and citron rootstock gives the oils a finer quality but there is no technical data that supports this claim [15].

According to Valerie Ann Worwood, bergamot is the main flavoring in Earl Gray Tea. It is also widely used in eau de cologne [16] and is also considered one of the most popular essential oils for use in perfumery.

There is an annual herb that is also called bergamot (*Monarda didyma*) but it is unrelated to bergamot essential oil. "FCF" indicates that the oil should be bergapten or furocoumarin-free (FCF).

1. **Class**: Esters, monoterpenes, and alcohol

2. **Family**: *Rutaceae*. This family of plants are commonly known at the citrus family. Species of the family generally have flowers that divide into four or five parts usually with a strong scent. They range in form and size from herbs to shrubs and large trees. The most common in this family include orange, lemon, lime and grapefruit.

3. **Distillation process**: Produced by cold expression from the peel of the nearly ripe fruit from the small bergamot tree (C. *bergamia*).

4. **Biochemical compounds**: Bergamot essential oil is primarily composed of monoterpene hydrocarbons, monoterpenes alcohols and esters. A typical chemical composition of bergamot is reported as follows:
   a. Monoterpenes: from 11 to 30%
   b. Alcohols: dihydrocuminic alcohol, (+)-linalool up to 14% (and negligible amounts of other alcohols)
   c. Esters: (-) linalyl acetate varies usually around 20% up to 60%
   d. Aldehydes: citrals
   e. Coumarins & furocoumarins: bergamotene, bergapten, bergaptol, auraptenol, limetin, byakangelicin, 5-geranoxy-7-methoxycoumarin

5. **Typical application/uses**:
   a. Analgesic
   b. Anthelmintic
   c. Antidepressant
   d. Anti-infectious
   e. Antibacterial especially for staphylococcus (pyogenic), meningitis, and streptococcus

f.   Antiseptic

g.   Antiparasitic

h.   Antispasmodic

i.   Antitoxic

j.   Antiviral

k.   Carminative

l.   Cicatrizant

m.   Cordially

n.   Diuretic

o.   Deodorant

p.   Digestive

q.   Expectorant

r.   Febrifuge

s.   Insecticide

t.   Laxative

u.   Rubefacient

v.   Stimulant (General)

w.   Sedative

x.   Stomachic

y.   Tonic

z.   Vermifuge

aa.   Vulnerary

6.   Chemical Composition:

    a.   Monoterpenes:

        i. α-pinene - 1.0%

        ii. β-pinene – 5.7%

        iii. β-bisabolene – 0.57%

        iv.   bergaptene - 0.23%

        v.   camphene – 4.0%

        vi.   d-limonene – up to 30%

    b.   Alcohols:

        i.   dihydrocuminic- alcohol, (+)-linalool – 13.45%

        ii.   nerol – 0.1%

        iii.   geraniol – 0.05%

        iv. α-terpineol – 0.13%

c. Esters:
    i. linalyl acetate – usually around 31.3% and up to 60%
    ii. nerol acetate – 0.42%
d. Aldehydes:
    i. citrals
e. Coumarins and furocoumarins: Remember, these compounds should be avoided for aromatherapy. Because bergapten, also known as 5-methoxypsoralen, (present in bergamot essential oils) has been shown to be phototoxic when tested on human skin. Since bergapten is phototoxic, it may increase DNA damage effects of ultraviolet light, although it can also protect against them. Bergapten is cytotoxic to the human hepatocellular carcinoma cell line; it kills cells directly, induces apoptosis, and inhibits proliferation [17].

7. **Systems:**
    a. Integumentary (skin hair, nails): Provides support and relief for acne, boils, oily skin, psoriasis, pruritus', scabies, eczema. Can also support healing for wounds, varicose veins, ulcers, seborrhea of skin and scalp. Makes an effective insect repellant. Bergamot has been found to inhibit the herpes simplex 1 virus, which causes cold sores. It is particularly effective with combination with tea tree and lavender for the treatment and relief of cold sores, chicken pox, and shingles.
    b. Respiratory: Serves as a pulmonary antiseptic, which provides support for chronic halitosis, sore throat, tonsilitis, colds, and flu
    c. Cardiovascular/lymphatic system: Provides relief and support for hemorrhoids
    d. Immune: Provides excellent support for colds and flu as well as general infections. May

support the immune system during shingles and chicken pox as well as malaria and yellow fever

    e.   Digestive: Provide support for painful digestion, dyspepsia, colitis, flatulence, and loss of appetite. Its action on the digestive system is carminative and useful in relieving colic and indigestion. Bergamot oil is particularly indicated for loss of appetite due to emotional stress.[13]

    f.   Genito-urinary/reproductive: because of its antiseptic properties, it may help with cystitis, leucorrhea, thrush, and has a nice tonic action on uterus challenges.

    g.   Central nervous system: This essential oil uplifts, balances, encourages and refreshes the entire body. It also helps sedate the thinking and depression along with stress related disorders. It cools anger, allays frustration and decreases sympathetic nervous system action. It is known to expand and open the hear chakra and aids in radiating love energy.

8. **Personality**: Bergamot personalities are fresh, caring, considerate, and full of energy. As they grow older, these individuals remain young at heart and have a joyful approach to life. Bergamot personalities enter the room smiling, bright, happy and in balance, at ease with the world and loving nature. These individuals are discriminating, tactful, practical, highly imaginative, caring and productive. Bergamot can see both sides of any issue which enables him/her to rebalance feelings and emotions.[18] Basil essential oil supports positive attributes: concentration and focus, confidence, balance, strength, joy, motivation, good cheer, and harmony. Bergamot oil can be used to counteract negative attributes: depression, anxiety, helplessness, apathy, bitterness, burnout, emptiness, exhaustion, grief, hopelessness, and emotional imbalances.[19]

9. **Safety**: Bergaptene is phototoxic on the skin, and sun exposure should be avoided after using bergamot during massage or in bath. The International Fragrance Research Association recommends that the amount of bergamot used in topical preparations should be limited to a maximum of 0.4 percent, except in bath preparations such as soaps and other bath preparations which are washed off the skin.[20] Dr. Scott Johnson states that bergamot may interfere with the enzymes responsible for drug metabolism of NSAIDs (non-steroidal anti-inflammatory drugs, including ibuprofen), proton-pump inhibitors, acetaminophen, antiepileptics, immune modulators, blood surge medications, blood pressure medications, antidepressants, antipsychotic and diabetic medications, antihistamines, antibiotics, and anesthetics.[21]

10. **Blending**: Top/middle note.

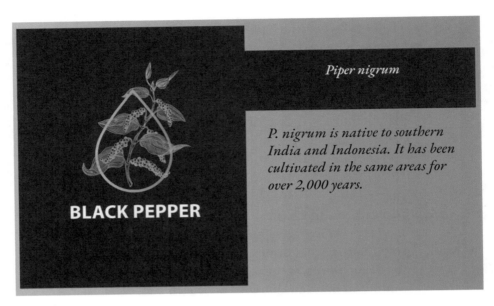

Piper nigrum

P. nigrum is native to southern India and Indonesia. It has been cultivated in the same areas for over 2,000 years.

Black Pepper
Piper nigrum

It is a perennial vine climbing to about 5 meters. The inflorescence is a pike of about 20 to 30 sessile flowers that do not mature simultaneously. When a few fruits are ripe, the spike is harvested. Ripe fruits are removed and allowed to ferment or are soaked in running water to remove the pericarps. The seeds are dried and powdered to give the white pepper of commence. Black peppers are more pungent and are produced from the unripe fruits on the harvested spikes. There are sun-dried, usually after soaking in hot water. The pungency is due to the presence of various resins and a yellow crystalline alkaloid called piperine.[22]

Pepper has been esteemed as a spice in India throughout recorded history and has been dispersed in trade throughout the world. Pepper was so important that the search for the source of the spice and the control of the trade was a significant factor influencing world exploration and history. Pepper is grown and harvested is mostly from India, Indonesia, and Madagascar.

1. **Class:** Sesquiterpenes, phenol ethers

2. **Family:** *Piperaceae*

3. **Distillation:** The essential oil of black pepper is produced by the steam distillation of the dried, but not quite ripe fruits of the pepper vine.

4. **Biochemicals**:
   a. Monoterpenes: (5%) α- & β-pinenes, thujene, camphene, sabinene, carene, limonene, phellandrene
   b. Sesquiterpenes: (approx. 89%) β-caryophyllene, α-humulene, α-gualene, α- & β-elemenes, β-bisabolene, calamenene
   c. Alcohols: terpinene-4-ol, α-terpineol, linalool, trans-pinocarveol, trans-carveol, phenol methyl-ethers: paracymene-8-ol, methyl carvacrol
   d. Ketones: dihydrocarvone
   e. Acetophenones: methyl acetophenones
   f. Aldehydes: piperonal
   g. Sulfur: n-formyl piperidine
   h. Acids: piperonylic

5. **Uses**:
   a. Analgesic
   b. Antiemetic
   c. Antimicrobial
   d. Aperitif
   e. Antiseptic
   f. Antispasmodic
   g. Aphrodisiac
   h. Bactericidal
   i. Carminative
   j. Diaphoretic
   k. Diuretic
   l. Expectorant
   m. Febrifuge
   n. Laxative
   o. Odontalgic
   p. Rubefacient
   q. Stimulant (CNS, glandular, and cardiovascular)
   r. Stomachic
   s. Tonic

6. **Chemical composition**: Black pepper is rich in monoterpene, hydrocarbons, and sesquiterpene hydrocarbons. The composition of black pepper can vary considerably according to origin and method of preparation. Monoterpene hydrocarbons are known for their analgesic, antiseptic, and tonic properties while sesquiterpene hydrocarbons may account for black pepper's antiviral properties. The greatest variation is within the monoterpene hydrocarbons groups as follows: [23]

   a. limonene: 0 – 40%
   b. β-pinene: 5 – 35%
   c. α-phellandrene: 1 – 27%
   d. β-phellandrene: 0 – 19%
   e. sabinene: 0 – 20%
   f. d-3-carene: trace to 15%
   g. myrcene: trace to 10%

   A typical chemical composition of black pepper is as follows: [23]

   a. α-pinene 5.8%
   b. camphene 0.1%
   c. β-pinene 10.4%
   d. d-3-carene 20.2%
   e. limonene 17.1%
   f. gamma-terpinene 0.2%
   g. para-cymene 0.8%
   h. terpinolene 1.0%
   i. d-elemene 2.5%
   j. α-copaene 2.3%
   k. β-elemene 0.4%
   l. β-caryophyllene 27.8%
   m. α-humulene 1.4%
   n. d-cadinene 0.8%
   o. caryophyllene oxide 0.6%

7. **Systems**:

   a. Integumentary (skin, nails, hair): Can provide support and healing for chilblains, bruises cuts, wounds, and dermatosis.

b. Respiratory: Support for catarrh, chronic bronchitis, laryngitis, and tonsillitis. Warms the body when feeling cold.

c. Muscular/skeletal: Provides support and relief of arthritis, muscle aches and pains, neuralgia, poor muscle tone, and temporary paralysis. May support and relieve stiffness and rheumatism.

d. Cardiovascular: Increases circulation (dilates capillaries to increase local blood flow)

e. Immune: Supports the body's defense against colds, flu, infections, and viruses. May provide support to reduce fever (body temperature).

f. Digestive: Supports liver function and stimulates liver-pancreas. Provides support for anemia, toothache, and tonsillitis. Increases saliva. May also help with reducing fats and stimulating appetite. For children and horses, it may provide support for colic. Supports digestion, constipation, diarrhea, flatulence, heartburn, nausea, and vomiting. Restores the colon for more natural function.

g. Genito-urinary/reproductive: Provides support and relief for frigidity and impotence. Stimulates kidney and urinary system. May increase urine flow and aid with detoxification.

h. Central nervous system: Serves as a mental stimulant and aids with alertness. It may also provide stamina to the body. It warms the soul, supporting and relieving indifference to life and it eases the stress from changes in life.

8. **Personality:** Black pepper is the older, sterner personality among the essential oils, but having said that, it can also be the livelier types of personality. They often seem older than their physical age, whether the baby whose eyes reflect deep wisdom or the 12-year-old who acts like a settled 42-year-old. This type of person will reprimand you for not having behaved correctly as at a social gathering —

particularly if you are a carefree Melissa type! These individuals can by extremely self-righteous (providing it suits them) and if allowed, may be dictatorial. On the other hand, they can be very loyal (if they like you). Black pepper essential oil supports positive attributes: comfort, stamina, endurance, motivation, and changeability. It counteracts negative attributes: emotional blockages, compulsions, confusion, disorientation, fatigue, begrudging, indecision, irrationality, anger, frustration, emotional coldness, apathy, and mental exhaustion.[24]

9. **Safety**: Black pepper oil is non-irritating and non-sensitizing, and there are no contraindications. Caution: there is always a possibility of irritation due to sensitivity with this oil, and it should always be diluted. Due to highly variable compositions and the possible dermatitis, it should be used with care in massage or bath.

10. **Blending**: Middle note.

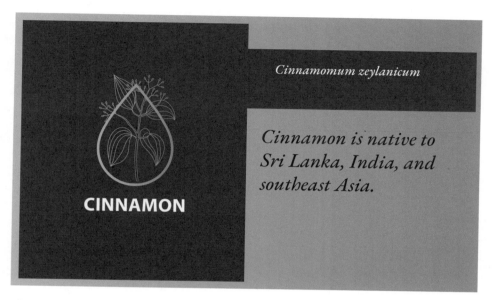

Cinnamomum zeylanicum

Cinnamon is native to Sri Lanka, India, and southeast Asia.

Cinnamon
Cinnamomum zeylanicum

Cinnamon produces the finest bark in sunny regions with an average temperature of 27 to 30 degrees Celsius. Cinnamon bark oil is a pale-yellow or brownish-yellowish liquid with an extremely powerful, diffusive, warm-spicy and tenacious odor. Cinnamon leaf (from the same plant) is a yellow to brownish yellow oil with a warm-spicy but rather harsh odor that lacks the rich body of the bark oil. It has some resemblance to the scent of clove leaf essential oil and clove stem essential oi.[25] The cinnamon bark essential oil can provide an effective remedy but must be used with caution as it is a severe dermal irritant and sensitizer.

Interestingly, cinnamon is often confused with cinnamon *cassia* (C. *cassia*) which is known as *cassia*. *Cassia* is sometimes referred to as Chinese cinnamon, false *cassia*. Both cassia and cinnamon have been used for several thousands of years in Eastern and Western cultures in treating chronic diarrhea, rheumatism, colds, abdominal and heart pains, kidney problems, hypertension, and female disorders such as amenorrhea and cramps. [26]

Cinnamon bark essential oil is used in pharmaceutical preparations as a carminative, stomachic, tonic or counterirritant and it is often included in mouth washes, liniments, nasal sprays, and toothpaste. Cinnamon leaf essential oil is used as a fragrance component of soaps, detergents, creams, lotions, and perfumes. [27]

A carbon dioxide extract of cinnamon bark at a 0.1% concentration completely suppressed the growth of numerous micro-organisms, including Escherichia coli – E. coli, Staphylococcus aureus – staph and Candida albicans – candida. Cinnamon bark oil was also found to have protein antifungal properties against fungi causing respiratory tract mycoses. [28]

Very interesting to note here that cinnamon bark essential oil is often adulterated with cassia, which is a coarser bark.

According to the work of Rolf Deininger as well as Pierre Franchomme and Daniel Penoel, cinnamon bark oil is effective against 98% of all pathogenic (+) gram and (-) gram bacteria. It is also effective against yeasts, candida, and fungi, including aspergillus, thereby preventing aflatoxin production. It is antiparasitic and prevents fermentation in the intestines. It is effect against diarrhea, colitis, amoebic dysentery enterotoxaemia, bacterial cystitis, and urinary infections with e. coli and tropical infections accompany by fever.[29]

1. **Class**: Aldehydes

2. **Family**: *Lauraceae*

3. **Distillation**: Cinnamon bark essential oil is obtained by steam or water distillation with cohobation. Cinnamon bark contains water-soluble volatile aromatic components, which can be recovered by extracting distillation water and adding the extract to water-distilled oils.

4. **Biochemical:**
    a. Monoterpenes: β-phellandrene, limonene, p-cymene
    b. Sesquiterpenes: β-caryophyllene
    c. Alcohols: 2-phenylethyl, cinnamic, benzyl alcohol, linalool, α-terpineol, borneol
    d. Esters: benzyl benzoate, 2-phenyl ethyl benzoate, methyl cinnamate, cinnamyl acetate (traces)
    e. Phenols: (up to 10%) eugenol, isoeugenol, phenol, 2-vinyl-phenol, camphor
    f. Aldehydes: cinnamaldehyde (>75%), hydroxy cinnamaldehyde, benzaldehyde, cumin aldehyde.
    g. Coumarin: coumarin >1%

Two sources for cinnamon essential oil are listed below, allowing a comparison of the different CO2 distillations. The oil sourced from Sri Lanka varies significantly in the CO2 distillation compared to the CO2 distillation sourced from Madagascar, particularly in the trans-cinnamon aldehyde. Oils are less expensive if produced using the CO2 extraction but may contain different cinnamic alcohol content depending on elevation and the natural temperature in sunny regions with an average temperature of 27 to 30 degrees Celsius. Plants harvested at this higher elevation will also provide a higher potency for prevention/treatment for antifungal and infection purposes.

- ❧ CO2 selective distillation: (sourced from Sri Lanka, cinnamon bark and leaf) 59% trans-cinnamon aldehyde, 10% cannula acetate, 2% eugenol, 1.7% 2-methoxy-cinnamon aldehyde, 1.3% cinnamic alcohol.
- ❧ CO2 total distillation: (sourced from Madagascar, cinnamon bark and leaf) 37% trans-cinnamon aldehyde, 3% cinnamic alcohol, 1.7% 2-methoxy cinnamon aldehyde, 0.4% eugenol, 0.15% coumarin.

With the differing properties based on extraction processes as well as the differing plant properties in these regions, the practitioner needs to fully research and confirm the source and composition of any cinnamon oils before using.[30]

5. **Uses:** Cinnamon leaf and bark oil, based on physical challenges:
    a. Antibacterial (large spectrum antibiotic)
    b. Anticoagulant (blood thinner)
    c. Anesthetic
    d. Antiodontalgic
    e. Antifungal
    f. Anti-infectious (intestinal, urinary)
    g. Antiparasitic
    h. Antiseptic
    i. Antimicrobial (one of the strongest agents, useful for resisting viral infections and contagious diseases)
    j. Antiputrefactive
    k. Antispasmodic
    l. Aphrodisiac
    m. Astringent
    n. Cardiac

o.   Carminative

p.   Emmenagogue

q.   Escharotic

r.   Germicidal

s.   Hemostatic

t.   Insecticide

u.   Stimulant

v.   Stomachic

w.   Sudorific

x.   Sonic (general, central nervous system, and reinforces uterine contractions)

y.   Vermifuge

6.   **Chemical Composition:** [31]

The typical composition of cinnamon is as follows:

Compound	Cinnamon Leaf	Cinnamon Bark
eugenol	80-96%	4-10%
eugenol acetate	1.0%	0.0
cinnamaldehyde	3.0%	40-50%
benzyl benzoate	3.0%	1.0%
α-pinene	0.0	0.2%
1,8 cineol	0.0	1.65%
linalool	0.0	2.3%
caryophyllene	0.0	1.35%

7.   **Systems:** Can be cinnamon bark or cinnamon leaf essential oils, based on the specific challenges of the patient; see Chapter 3 for greater explanation of interactions with body systems:

a.   Integumentary (skin, hair, nails): Excellent support to relieve candida as well as foot fungus and warts. Supports relief from head lice and scabies. Supports the body from insect bites and stings. Tightens loose tissues; however, as a dermal irritant, avoid use on sensitive or damaged skin. For any topical application, use only if very diluted (1 to 3 percent).

b. Muscular/skeletal: Serves as a respiratory tonic and stimulant. Antiseptic when inhaled and could actually ease colds and breathing along with bronchitis, pleurisy. Raises body temperature.

c. Cardiovascular: In low dosages, eases muscular spasm and rheumatic pain.

d. Immune: As one of the strongest antibacterial agents, provides excellent support for resisting viral infections and contagious diseases. Also provides support to fight tropical infections and fevers.

e. Digestive: Provides support to relieve and eliminate pyorrhea (a gum disease). Provides support for toothaches as an anesthetic. When diluted properly, internal use includes intestinal infection, gut parasites (amoebas, amoebic cysts, spasms). Supports asthenia – loss of tone, dyspepsia, colitis, gas, nausea, vomiting, and pancreas function. May support digestion and peristalsis of large intestines with respect to constipation, diarrhea. Provides stimulation and support for digestive complaints including inflammation from colitis.

f. Genito-urinary/reproductive: May induce menstruation, eases period pain, and regulates scanty menstruation. During birth, supports uterine contractions and helps with postpartum depression. Provides support for kidney problems, cystitis, urinary infections, and vaginitis. Also provides support for male impotence and frigidity.

g. Central nervous system: When inhaled, provides warming of body (physically) and mind (psychically). Provides support for anemia, insomnia, debility, nervous depression, exhaustion and feelings of weakness and depression. Provides relief from emotional coldness and isolation and may release fear. Arouses senses and stimulates the psychic digestion (emotional and mental processing).

8. **Personality**: Cinnamon is the larger-than-life, affable type of person — practical and intelligent with a strong personality. They can be very conservative in thought and nature, preferring the comfort of the establishment rather than risking the discomfort of the unknown. They do enjoy a bit of excitement now and again, providing it doesn't interfere with their well-being. Individuals with a cinnamon character are warming, secular, and fair minded. Cinnamon oil supports these positive attributes: invigorated, steadfast, benevolent, strength of character, practical, energized, realistic, and direct. Cinnamon essential oil is used to counteract these negative attributes: instability, severity, bleakness, malice, spitefulness, coldness, fear, nervous exhaustion, debility, introversion, superficiality.[32]

9. **Safety**: Cinnamon bark essential oils are confirmed dermal irritant and sensitizer, with a higher cinnamaldehyde content. Cinnamic aldehyde is easily absorbed into skin and can cross react with apery balsam. It should be used in a highly diluted form and for local application only.

   ♠ *Caution: avoid during early pregnancy.*
   ♠ *Caution: avoid during gastrointestinal ulcers.*

   According to Kurt Schnaubelt, cinnamon bark and leaf provoke skin sensitization in approximately 5% of the population when applied topically.[33] These oils are preferably used internally, which is less problematic.

10. **Blending**: Base note.

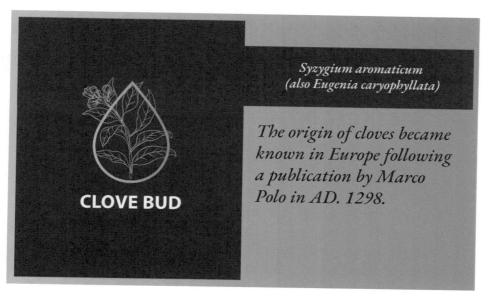

Syzygium aromaticum (also Eugenia caryophyllata)

The origin of cloves became known in Europe following a publication by Marco Polo in AD. 1298.

CLOVE BUD

Clove Bud
Syzygium aromaticum (also Eugenia caryophyllata)

To a knowledgeable practitioner who is familiar with essential oils, clove falls into the category of the "spicies" essential oils (other categories include "leafies" "greenies" and "rooties" "seedies" "fruities" "herbies" and "resinies"). "Spicies" are defined as essential oils that are extracted from various parts of plant or trees commonly known as "spicies." These oils include cinnamon, clove, nutmeg, turmeric, etc. The clove tree, primarily grown in Madagascar, is a long-lived tree reported to remain productive for 150 yrs.[34] It is an evergreen tree that grows up to 15 meters high with glossy green leaves, fragrant red flowers, and purple fruit. Cloves were introduced to Zanzibar in the 19th century. Zanzibar, now part of Tanzania, has become the world's largest exporter of cloves.

The modern English name of clove is from the French "clou", meaning nail, derived from the Latin "clavus." The first recorded use was in the Chinese Han period 220-206 BC where it was used to "sweeten the breath."[35]

The clove bud essential oil is a clear to yellow mobile liquid, become brown with a strong, sweet, and spicy odor. The clove leaf essential oil is a dark-brown mobile liquid with a harsh woody, phenolic, slightly sweet aroma. The clove leaf essential oil is often rectified and is usually a pale-yellow color with a sweeter, less harsh, dry woody odor, closer to that of eugenol.

Adulterants of clove bud essential oil are usually clove stem or clove leaf and/or clove terpenes remaining after eugenol extractions.[36]

Clove essential oil has been used as a local analgesic for the relief of toothache. Eugenol, like other phenols, acts to depress sensory receptors involved in pain perception. It has antiviral and antifungal effects. Essential oil from clove has an impressive range of action against pathogens, and illness of all kinds. It is antiparasitic and works for gum infections toothaches and tonsilitis. Research indicates its usefulness for poliomyelitis, multiple sclerosis, tuberculosis, cholera Hodgkin's disease, hepatitis, malaria, viral colitis, dysentery, amoebas, spasmodic colitis, thyroid imbalances, arthritis, viral neuritis, neuralgia, salpingitis and cystitis. Dr. Schnaubelt preferred mode of use is internally only unless highly diluted.[37]

1. **Class**: Phenol, esters

2. **Family**: *Myrtaceae*

3. **Distillation**: Clove bud essential oil is water-distilled from the dried flower buds of *S. aromaticum*. The clove buds are mashed prior to distillation. If the cloves are steam-distilled, hydrolysis takes place, and most of the natural acetyl eugenol is converted to eugenol. Compared to steam distillation, the level of hydrolysis that occurs during water distillation is minimal. The eugenol content of water distillation is typically 85-90%, while the eugenol content of steam distilled clove bud essential oil is typically 91-95%

4. **Biochemical**:
   a. Phenols: eugenol (up to 85% - lesser amount than stem or leaf) chavicol, 4-allylphenol
   b. Esters: (22%): eugenyl acetate, benzyl, terpinene-4-ol, and ethyl phenyl acetates: trace

of methyl salicylate

c. Sesquiterpenes: (up to 6%) α- & β-caryophyllene, α- & β-humulene, α-amorphene, α-muurolene, calamenene, calacorene, pinene

d. Oxides: (<3%): caryophyllene oxide, humulene oxide also benzylic acid, traces of vanillin, furfurol, acetyl eugenol

e. CO_2 selective: eugenol, eugenyl acetate, caryophyllene

f. Stem: eugenol, eugenyl acetate, methyl salicylate, caryophyllene, pinene, furfurol

g. Leaf: less eugenol than stem, little or no eugenyl acetate, other minor constituents

5. **Uses:**
   a. Analgesic
   b. Anthelmintic
   c. Antiemetic
   d. Antihistamine
   e. Antioxidant
   f. Antiseptic
   g. Antifungal
   h. Anti-infectious
   i. Antibacterial (powerful large spectrum, pyogenes var. aureus, e coli, proteus, strep)
   j. Antiparasitic
   k. Antispasmodic
   l. Antiviral
   m. Aphrodisiac
   n. Carminative
   o. Cicatrizant
   p. Expectorant
   q. Larvicidal
   r. Parturient
   s. Spasmolytic
   t. Splenetic
   u. Stomachic
   v. Sonic (uterine, nervous, hypertension)
   w. Vermifuge

6. **Chemical Composition**: The typical composition of the clove bud, clove stem and clove leaf are: [36]

Compound	Clove Leaf	Clove Stem	Clove Bud
eugenol	85-90%	87-92%	80-85%
eugenyl acetate	0-10%	3-3.5%	8-12%
isoeugenol	-	Trace	-
caryophyllene	10-15%	6-8%	6-10%
isocaryophyllene	-	-	0-2.0%

7. **Systems**:
   a. Integumentary (skin, hair, nails): Provides excellent support for acne, cuts and skin parasites, scabies, fungal infections, athletes foot: May help with bruising, warts, herpes, shingles and prickly heat. Also serves as an effective mosquito repellant; however, should only be used in a highly diluted form on skin (less than 1 percent)
   b. Respiratory: Provides support for asthma, sinusitis, and bronchitis. Works especially well to support pulmonary afflictions.
   c. Muscular/skeletal: Provides support for rheumatoid arthritis, rheumatism, and sprains. Very useful in polio when combined with mustard and used as a plaster
   d. Cardiovascular: Provides support for hypotension, acts as a circulatory stimulant.
   e. Immune: Provides support for colds, flu, and minor infections and supports prevention of infections. Also provides support for malaria and viral infections. Useful with shingles and herpes, and to provide support for multiple sclerosis and Hodgkin's disease
   f. Digestive: Provides excellent support for toothaches, dental infections, tonsillitis, viral

hepatitis, intestinal virus, bacterial otitis, cholera, dysentery (amebic) colic spasms, dyspepsia, and nausea. Also provides support for intestinal intoxications and fermentation and parasites. Stimulates appetite and digestion.

g.   Genito-urinary/reproductive: Acts as an aphrodisiac and works well with impotence/ frigidity. May ease childbirth by easing anxiety and increasing relaxation during inhalation.

h.   Central nervous system: Provides support for general debility and fatigue. Stimulates the mind and memory. It uplifts depression, lethargy, tension, and headaches. It may help with fatigue, asthenia (on the physical and intellectual aspect) and combats drowsiness.

8.   **Personality**: According to Salvator Battaglia[38], the clove bud personality is imbued with the rich spicy aroma of clove oil, suggesting that the individual is dynamic, self-assured, and full of energy. Valerie Worwood uses clove essential oil to create positive states of contentment, creativity, focus, happiness, and self-awareness.[39] Clove bud essential oils support emotional healing of expressed, unrealized anger. It can also provide support for dementia, and general feelings of misery, pain, quarrelsomeness, and worthlessness.[40]

9.   **Safety**: At high dosages (0.5 mL/kg) clove bud essential oil is toxic. A near-fatal ingestion of clove oil was reported involving a 2-year-old boy who had drunk between 5-10 ml of clove oil.[41]

   ♠ Caution: clove bud essential oil, especially in young children, causes central nervous system depression, hepatic necrosis, convulsions and/or major hemostatic abnormalities.

   ♠ Caution: It has been reported to be a potential skin irritant and sensitizing agent.

Clove oil should be used in less than 1 percent dilution, as it may cause dermatitis. Clove bud essential oil is slightly less hazardous than stem or leaf.

10. **Blending**: Base note.

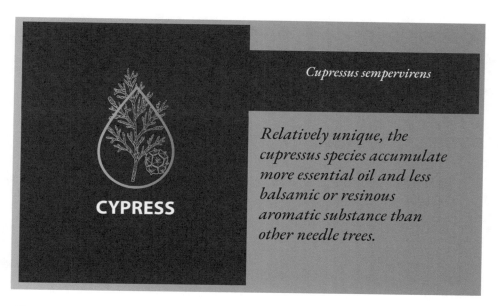

Cupressus sempervirens

Relatively unique, the cupressus species accumulate more essential oil and less balsamic or resinous aromatic substance than other needle trees.

Cypress
Cupressus sempervirens

The tree originates in the eastern Mediterranean countries and can be found along the coast of southern France, Italy, Corsica, Sardinia, Sicily North Africa, Spain, Portugal and the Balkan countries. Most of the oil is distilled in southern France. It is an extremely old species dating back to the Pliocene era (5.3 to 18 million years). It is exceptionally long-lived, and some trees are believed to be two thousand years old.[42]

The oils of *cupressus* needles contain monoterpenes, sesquiterpenes, and diterpenes, and the wood oil contains thymol and carvacrol. With the current trend toward esotericism in aromatherapy, it is surprising that there is not yet a range of prehistoric aromatic on the market.[43]

According to Kurt Schnaubelt, the effects of cypress cannot be attributed to any of the main constituents. An evaluation of essential oils according to their dominant synergy is therefore a rather simplistic way to assess the more obvious pharmacological effect of these substances. However, the possible generalization is still very useful. The finer or deeper effects of oils still have to be evaluated individually, which throws the modern aromatherapy user back to old-fashioned empiricism—gaining knowledge through carefully documented experience and experiments.[44]

Essential oil of cypress derives its multiple uses from all of its components. It is useful for all bronchial complaints, and it is a choice spasmolytic for whooping cough. Aromatherapy recommends cypress for lung diseases like tuberculosis and pleurisy (in conjunction with *Myrtis communis*). It is a decongestant for prostate, veins, and the lymphatic system. Its bitter principles strengthen a weak pancreas. It is an intestinal and neuro-tonic. It helps to prevent the spread of varicose veins, hemorrhoids, and edema, especially of the lower limbs. Dr. Schnaubelt's preferred mode of use in Internal and topical and he mentions that the quality of this oil is often uncertain.[45]

1. **Class**: Monoterpenes

2. **Family**: *Cupressaceae*

3. **Distillation**: Cypress essential oil is steam-distilled from the leaves (needles) and twigs of *C. sempervirens* obtained by pruning the trees in autumn

4. **Biochemical**:
    a. monoterpenes: α-pinene (>55%), -3-carene (>30%), limonene, terpinolene, sabinene, β-pinene
    b. sesquiterpenes: α-cedrene, & cadinene
    c. sesquiterpenols: cedrol (7%), a-cadinol
    d. monoterpenols: terpinene-4-ol, α-terpineol, borneol,
    e. diterpenols (labdanic): manool, sempervirol
    f. diterpenic acids: neocupressic acid
    g. ester: a-terpinyl acetate
    h. also: α-methyl-ether, (terpineol methyl-ether) and ketones (thujone) in variable quantities, depending on type

5. **Uses:**
    a. Antirheumatic
    b. Antiseptic
    c. Anti-infectious
    d. Antibacterial

    e.   Antimycobacterial
    f.   Antispasmodic
    g.   Astringent
    h.   Deodorant
    i.   Decongestant (lymphatic, prostatic)
    j.   Diuretic
    k.   Emmenagogue
    l.   Hepatic
    m.   Mucolytic
    n.   Hemostatic (styptic)
    o.   Styptic
    p.   Sudorific (regulator)
    q.   Tonic (neuro and intestinal)
    r.   Vasoconstrictive
    s.   Venous

6. **Chemical Composition**: A typical chemical composition of cypress is reported as follows: [38]
    a. α-pinene 20.4%
    b.   camphene 3.6%
    c.   sabinene 2.8%
    d. β-pinene 2.9%
    e.   8-3-carene 21.5%
    f.   myrcene and α-terpinene 1.1%
    g.   terpinolene 6.3%
    h.   linalool 0.07%
    i.   bornyl acetate 0.3%
    j.   cedrol 5.35%
    k.   cadinene 1.7%

7. **Systems**:
    a.   Integumentary: Provides excellent support for mature skin as well as relief for oil and acne skin. Supports skin that is over hydrated including excessive perspiration. Also provides support for edema (simple water retention), varicose veins, and wound healing. Stimulates skin circulation

b. Respiratory: Provides relief for sore throat, hoarseness, and laryngitis sinusitis. Provides support for asthma, bronchitis, spasmodic cough, whooping cough, and pleurisy.

c. Muscular/skeletal: Relieves muscle cramps. Aids arthritis and rheumatism.

d. Cardiovascular: May support poor circulation, hemorrhoids (internal and external) and varicosities. Supports blood purification.

e. Immune: Stimulates the immune system.

f. Digestive: Excellent support for bleeding gums, colitis, and gut infections. Stimulates sluggish intestines and hepato-pancreatic function.

g. Endocrine: Serves as a female stimulant. May also increase pancreatic action.

h. Genito-urinary/reproductive: Induces menstruation, eases painful periods, menopausal hot flashes, and tension. May provide relief from cramps and PMS because it regulates menstrual cycle. Also decongests the prostate. Increases urine flow, eases edema (simple water retention) and provides support for enuresis (bed wetting).

i. Central nervous system: Excellent support for nervous tension, stress-related conditions. Provides relief for debility, asthenia, anger, lack of concentration, sexual preoccupation, nervous breakdown, uncontrolled crying and selfishness. Provides balance for someone who steals and wastes mental and physical energy or money from others. Provides a beautiful spiritual aid for transition. Cleanses the spirit and removes psychic blocks.

8. **Personality**: People perceive cypress personalities to be powerful and able to sort out most problems. If they are not a person's first choice of confidant, it is perhaps because they see them as proud and even arrogant. This

is because of their air of honesty, lawlessness, and their unbending search for truth.[46]

The character of cypress is protective, righteous, wise, and loves clear guidance in life. Valerie Worwood recommends this essential oil be used for strength, comfort, change and direction in life, assertion, control, understanding, balance, wisdom, purity of heart, willpower, and being straightforward. She also suggests to use cypress essential oil to counteract these negative attributes: grief, sorrow, self-loathing, being dominated, opinionated, jealous, weal-willed, unable to speak up for oneself, emotionally tired, lack of concentration, absentminded and uncontrollable passions.[46] These personalities make wonderful parents and grandparents by establishing clear boundaries that allow children to feel comfortable in their presence, while encouraging the children's free spirits. Phillippe Mailhebiau describes the cypress personality: "The splendor of the cypress a fine slender tree rising like a flame towards the starry, endless sky, represents the sacred flame of life, the unchangeable, eternal essence, and powerfully evokes the spiritual archetype of cypress, a tall, fine-looking old man with the wisdom granted by a thousand years of intense, disciplined life." [48]

9. **Safety**: Tested at low dose non-toxic, non-irritant and non-sensitizing. The wood from the tree presents possible contact dermatitis (not the essential oil). Should be avoided during pregnancy and for clients with high blood pressure. Should not be used with cancers, uterine and breast fibrosis.

10. **Blending**: Middle/base note.

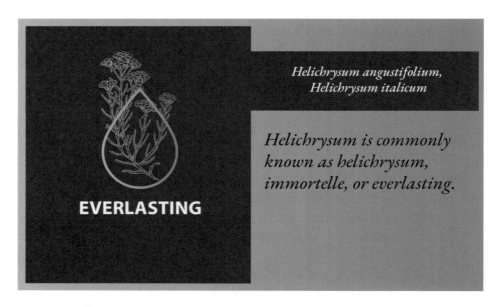

Helichrysum angustifolium,
Helichrysum italicum

Helichrysum is commonly known as helichrysum, immortelle, or everlasting.

Everlasting
Helichrysum angustifolium, Helichrysum italicum

In the Netherlands, it is also known as strawflower. This plant is a strongly aromatic shrub with many branched stems that are woody at the base, and it grows up to 0.6 meters high. When dried, these beautiful, brightly colored, and shapely like daisy flowers last "forever;" therefore, the common names everlasting or immortelle are quite appropriate to the plant. The plant grows wild in the Mediterranean climate, and fields to produce essential oils are cultivated in the south of France, Italy, former Yugoslavia, and other Mediterranean countries.

Helichrysum oil provides superior antihematoma and skin regenerating activity. Additional benefits include regulating cholesterol and stimulating liver cells. *Helichrysum* oil is an excellent mucolytic and an effective free-radical scavenger, protecting newly formed cells. Dr. Schnaubelt's preferred mode of use is typically only internally in low dosages, combined with lemon and rosemary verbenone to stimulate detoxification. When using high quality, unadulterated oils from confirmed suppliers, the aromatherapy usage is authentic and effective [49].

Approximately 500 species of *helichrysum* exist, but many of these do not produce essential oil. The main species used for production of essential oil include [50]:

H. angustifolium	Corsica and former Yugoslavia
H. stoechas DC	France
H. gymnocephalum	Madagascar
H. patulum	South Africa

1. **Class**: Monoterpenoid, ester

2. **Family**: *Compositae* or *Asteraceae*

3. **Distillation**: *Helichrysum angustifolium* is steam distilled for the flowering tops

4. **Biochemical**: Listed below are the constituents from *H. angustifolium*, harvested in Yugoslavia:
    a. Terpenes: limonene, pinene y-curcumene
    b. Alcohols: nerol, geraniol, linalool, furfurol
    c. Aldehyde: isovaleric
    d. Esters: neryl acetate
    e. Phenol: eugenol
    f. Ketones: 3,5 dimethyloctane-4,6-dione; 2,4-dimenthylheptane-3,5-dione.
    g. *Note here: Yugoslavian is less rich than the French (H. stoechas) in esters, alcohols, carbonyl compounds and rich in acids.

5. **Uses**:
    a. Antiallergenic
    b. Antihistamine
    c. Anti-inflammatory
    d. Antimicrobial
    e. Antiphlogistic
    f. Antispasmodic
    g. Antitussive
    h. Antiseptic
    i. Astringent

      j.   Antihematoma (anticoagulant)
      k.   Emollient
      l.   Expectorant
      m.   Eungicidal
      n.   Hepatic
      o.   Anti-hypercholesterol
      p.   Mucolytic
      q.   Rervine
      r.   Splenic
      s.   Sedative

6. **Chemical Composition**: A typical composition of everlasting essential oil contains 30 to 50 percent of nerol and neryl acetate [51]:
   a. α-pinene
   b. β-pinene
   c. myrcene
   d. limonene
   e. 1,8 cineol
   f. borneol
   g. linalool
   h. 4,7-dimetyl-6-octen-3-one
   i. several diketones: 3,5 dimethyloctane-4,6-dione
   j. 2,4-dimethylheptane-3,5-dione

7. **Systems**:
   a. **Integumentary**: Provides excellent support for traumas, bruises, (internal and external), burns, acne, allergies, dermatitis, eczema. It supports regenerating as it stimulates new cells. It aids broken veins, stretch marks, inflammation, spots, warts, wounds, old scars.
   b. **Respiratory**: Provides support for asthma, bronchitis, sinusitis, spasmodic and chronic coughs and whooping coughs.
   c. **Muscular/skeletal**: Provides relief from muscular aches and pains, arthritis, rheumatism,

sprains, strained muscles. Also provides support for plantar fasciitis and Dupuytren contracture.

d.   **Cardiovascular**: Regulates blood pressure and cleanses and thins blood. Aids varicosities hematomas, as well as internal and external phlebitis.

e.   Increases arterial and venous circulation and increases lymphatic drainage. Supports detoxification.

f.   **Immune**: Provides support for bacterial and viral infections. Also supports body functions during colds, flu, candida, and allergies. Serves as an antiviral for herpes.

g.   **Digestive**: Provides support for liver congestion or fatigue and even headache from liver congestions. Supports viral colitis, regulates pancreas and gall bladder (bile) secretion. Provides support for spleen congestion. Also supports detoxification from drugs, especially nicotine. Serves as a liver stimulant and works well with rosemary verbenone, and lemon.

h.   **Genito-urinary/reproductive**: Provides support for cystitis, herpes, Bartholinitis (inflamed glands around the vaginal area).

i.   **Central nervous system**: Excellent support for depression, debility nervous exhaustion. Provides relief for headaches resulting from liver congestion, migraines, neuralgia, stress related conditions, and shock phobias. Improves meridian flow.

8.   **Personality**: The everlasting (also known as *immortelle*) profile is one of quietness, introversion, and youth, with a quiet knowledge that comes from inner connections to the spirituality of our world and the understanding that there are greater things in heaven and earth than we can see. The immortelle personality is highly spiritually evolved and often seem almost fair-like with a high

consciousness and mental agility. They will forgive quickly, do not bear grudges, and will not encourage the company of anyone who commits wrongs against them or others. Their character is gentleness, harmonizing, caring, warming and meditative. This oil encourages the positive attributes of acceptance of change, positive dreams, energy, patience, idealism, perseverance, inner strength and (positive) inner child. This beautiful oil counteracts negative attributes of stress, tension, emotional crisis, depression, mental and emotional exhaustion, insecurity, hyper-sensitivity, grief, addiction, (negative) inner child, and physical, emotional, and mental abuse [52].

9.   **Safety**: Tested as non-toxic, non-irritant, non-sensitizing. Absolute: non-irritating and non-sensitizing as well as non-phototoxic. Avoid with anticoagulant medications due to the possibility of hemorrhage.

10. **Blending**: Base note.

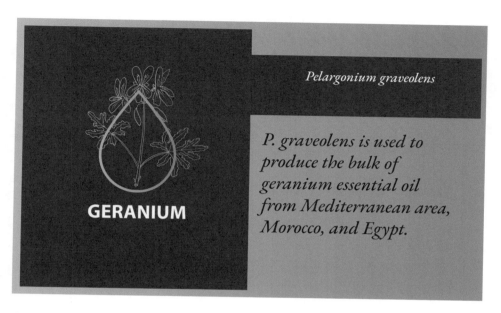

Pelargonium graveolens

P. graveolens is used to produce the bulk of geranium essential oil from Mediterranean area, Morocco, and Egypt.

GERANIUM

Geranium
Pelargonium graveolens

China's geranium essential oil produces high yield, although not as sweet. Many forms, varieties, and hybrids of the Pelargonium species exist around the world and are used to produce various types of geranium essential oils. The main species used for essential oils:

- *P. graveolens*
- *P. capitatum*
- *P. capitatum x radens*
- *P. odoratissimum*

Bourbon geranium is produced from the cultivar rose, which is a hybrid of *P. capitatum* and *P. capitatum x radens,* commonly known as *P. graveolens*.

Historical research into the origins of geranium plants can be confusing, considering that there are more than 250 natural species of Pelargonium. This beautiful plant is a perennial, shrubby, hairy plant that grows up to 1 meter in height with fragrant blooms. The first geranium plants grown for the French perfume industry were planted in Algeria in 1847. In the 1880s, extensive plantations were established in Reunion islands. Geranium oil is also produced in other parts of the world, such as China and Egypt. The Chinese geranium is very similar to bourbon, while Egypt geranium is quite different. The number of geraniums which are produced and available are usually distinguished by a country of origin with prefix: Reunion, Chinese, Egyptian or Moroccan [53].

The first reference to geranium is in Pedanius Dioscorides "Materia Medica" from the Greek *geranos*, a crane, because of the shape of the long beaked fruit. The plant and its fragrant leaves were used by the Romans [54].

Contradictory applications and confusion over the therapeutic activity of geranium oil may occur when researching proper wellness support using the essential oil. This confusion originates from transcribing Culpeppers' and other herbal texts which refer only to *G. robertianium* which has a complete different chemical composition to the geranium oil produced commercially today. [55]

1. **Class**: Alcohol, ester, and ketone

2. **Family**: *Geraniaceae*

3. **Distillation**: Geranium is steam-distilled from the leaves and branches of *P. graveolens*.

4. **Biochemical**:
    a. Monoterpenes: α- & β-phellandrene
    b. Sesquiterpenes: (+)α-copaene, d- & y-cadinenes (-)-4-guaialadiene-6-9, α- & β-bourbonenes, guaiazulene
    c. Alcohols: β-phenyl ethylic alcohol
    d. Monoterpene alcohols: (approx. 65%): (-) linalool, α-terpineol, (-)-citronellol (>32%), geraniol (>23%), nerol, menthol
    e. Sesquiterpenes: 10-epi-y-eudesmol (found in P. odoratissimum only)
    f. Esters (approx. 35%): citronellyl formate (>14%), geranyl, linalyl formates: citronellyl & geranyl acetate, citronellyl, geranyl, phenylethyl tiglates, citronellyl, geranyl propionates, citronellyl, and geranyl butyrates.

g. Oxides: 1,8 cineol, cis- and trans-rose oxide, cis- & trans-linalool oxide.

h. Aldehydes: neral, geranial, citronellal

i. Ketone: methyl heptenone, menthone, isomenthone (>8%) piperitone, 11-nor-bourbonanone

j. Sulfur: dimethyl sulfide

k. Nitrogen: citronellyl diethylamide

5. Uses:
   a. antidepressant
   b. antihemorrhagic
   c. anti-inflammatory
   d. anti-infectious
   e. antiseptic
   f. antibacterial
   g. antifungal
   h. analgesic
   i. antispasmodic
   j. astringent
   k. cicatrizant
   l. cytophylactic
   m. diuretic
   n. deodorant
   o. hemostatic
   p. hepatic stimulant
   q. styptic
   r. tonic
   s. vermifuge
   t. vulnerary

6. **Chemical composition**: Chemical composition of geranium essential oil from different places of origins varies greatly as seen in the chart below:

Constituent	Bourbon	Chinese	Egypt
linalool	12.90%	3.96%	9.47%
citronellol	21.28%	40.23%	27.40%
nerol	1.24%	0.67%	0.88%
geraniol	17.45%	6.45%	18.0%
citronellyl formate	8.37%	11.35%	6.74%
geranyl formate	7.55%	1.92%	4.75%
geranyl butyrate	1.34%	0.98%	1.48%
geranyl tiglate	1.04%	1.32%	1.06%
isomenthone	7.20%	5.70%	5.39%
guaia-6,9-diene	3.90%	4.40%	0.27%

Battaglia[56]

7. **Systems**:

    a.   Integumentary: Provides support for various skin conditions including acne, burns, bruises, broken capillaries. Provides relief for oily skin (balances oil grand secretion) and works well on congested and mature skin. Supports the body's fight against dermatitis, fungus, ulcers, eczema, lice, ringworm. May act as a mosquito repellant. Supports cellular regeneration and wound healing, especially after facial or plastic surgery. Excellent support for lymphatic drainage with comfrey and arnica extracts and especially helichrysum.

    b.   Respiratory: Provides support for sore throat, tonsilitis, and asthma Helps clear excessive mucus.

    c.   Muscular/skeletal: Supports rheumatism and osteoarthritis.

    d.   Cardiovascular: Serves as a wonderful circulatory tonic and aids poor circulation. Also provides relief of hemorrhoids, hemorrhoidal itching, and phlebitis. Offers anti-coagulant properties and stimulates lymphatic system.

e. Immune: Serves as a stimulant for the immune system.

f. Digestive: Possible internal uses include jaundice, gastritis, and colitis. Cleanses digestive system of mucus and serves as a liver tonic. It may work as an essential oil to help gastric ulcers and enterocolitis as an abdomen rub on the organs.

g. Endocrine: May work with adrenal, cortical and glandular challenges.

h. Genito-urinary/reproductive: Provides support during menopause and PMS and relieves engorgement of breasts. The oil can be combined with synergetic herbs providing aromatic medicine and applied as a paste across the chest. Also works as a kidney tonic, diuretic.

i. Central nervous system: Provides support with neuro-balancing, nervous tension, neuralgia, and stress problems. Acts as a sedative. Serves as an antidepressant by quelling anxiety, reducing stress, and uplifting emotions

8. **Personality**: The geranium personality is friendly and comforting, not in any way extroverted or overly talkative. These personalities are "mothering," always taking care of someone or something. Geranium personalities move forward in life while avoiding drama and noise. They allow others the freedom to have their own thoughts, and never interfere unless asked to help—which can be infuriating if you don't have the courage to ask. Geranium is a warm, kind, and generous personality who deserves to be appreciated for who they are. [57] Their character is balancing, healing, uplifting, and comforting. Geranium essential oil can be used to encourage these positive attributes: consolation, solace, adjustment, regeneration, honor, friendlessness, mothering, stability, and steadiness. It can also be used to counteract these negative attributes: anxiety, depression, acute fear, extreme moods, confusion, rigidity,

instability, moodiness, lack of self-esteem, overwhelming emotions, crisis, aggression, irrationality, discontent, worry, and heartache [58].

9. **Safety:** Absolute tested at low dose. Low toxic, non-irritant, generally non-sensitizing. Avoid during early pregnancy. According to Len and Shirley Price, this beautiful essential oil is to be used with care on the skin of hypertensive individuals. Thirty-two scented leaf, Pelargonium essential oils were testing in vitro and found to be spasmolytic [59].

10. **Blending**: Middle note.

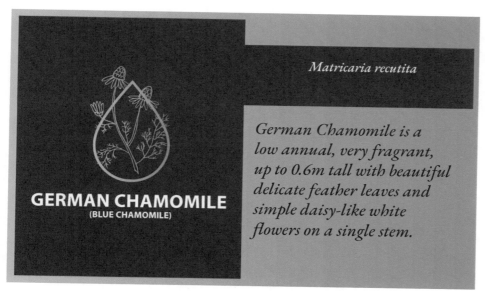

Matricaria recutita

German Chamomile is a low annual, very fragrant, up to 0.6m tall with beautiful delicate feather leaves and simple daisy-like white flowers on a single stem.

German Chamomile (Blue Chamomile)
Matricaria recutita

It is native to Europe, particularly in central and northern Europe. Plants are cultivated in Hungary, former Yugoslavia, Bulgaria, Russia, Germany, Belgium, and Spain. Hungary is one of the main producers of the essential oil.

This beautiful aromatic oil is deep, ink-colored blue with an intensely sweet scent. Sometimes, the pure, undiluted oil has an intense aroma that many people find overwhelming and unpleasant, especially compared to the Roman chamomile.

According to Kurt Schnaubelt, essential oil chemical constituents occurring in the plants naturally exhibit subtle differences from laboratory synthesized molecules. The naturally occurring oils often exhibit healing properties with more robust activity than the synthetic counterparts. Usually, the essential oil component is a pure enantiomer (mirror images that are not superimposable). One example of superior biological activity tied to the biological occurring enantiomer is the essential oil produced from German chamomile. Only the natural oil with the enantiomer pure (-)α-bisabolol, displays truly impressive anti-inflammatory qualities. Synthetic bisabolol is not enantiomerically pure but a racemic mixture of both enantiomers, which is distinctly less effective [60].

Matricaria recutita is one of the most reliable anti-inflammative agents in aromatherapy. However, its capability to neutralize toxic bacterial metabolic wastes, which are often the cause of fever during acute illnesses, is often overlooked. Dr. Schnaubelt's recommended application includes both external and internal for reliable qualities. Commercially available oils are often the less effective bisabolol oxide or bisabolon types, which contain little or no (-)α-bisabolol. German chamomile oils show a great variation in price, illustrating the extensive industrial adulteration of the essential oil [61].

Sylla Sheppard-Hanger cautions that the essential oil should not be confused with Tanacetum annuum called "wild", "blue" or "atlas" chamomile [62].

1. **Class**: Sesquiterpenols, sesquiterpene

2. **Family**: *Compositea* or *Asteraceae*

3. **Distillation**: German chamomile essential oil is steam-distilled from the dried flower heads. The essential oil content is highest at the beginning of flowering. Drying the flowers at 40 to 45 degrees C is reported to preserve the matricarin, and the resulting essential oil is reputed to contain the highest potency. [63]

4. **Biochemical**:
    a. Sesquiterpenes: chamazulene, dihydro-chamazulene I and II, bisabolenes, trans- β-farnesene
    b. Alcohols: (-) +α-bisabolol 8%, spathulenol, farnesol
    c. Oxides: bisabol oxides (>24%), β & C, epoxy bisabolol
    d. Coumarins: umbelliferon, herniarin
    e. Lactones: trans-en-in-dicyclo-ether

The CO2 extract (select) 38% steam volatile components, bisabolol 6%, matricin 2.8%. This is not degraded to blue chamazulene (latter has 1/10th anti-inflammatory activity).

CO2 extract (total) has full contact of proazulenes (matricin – this is not degraded to blue chamazulene as the latter has 1/10th anti-inflammatory activity). It also contains bisabolol, bisabolol oxide, cis and trans-en-in-dicyclo-ether, spathulenol and other guajanolides, herniarin and coumarin, flavone (apigenin), and cuticular waxes[64].

5. **Uses**: Many of these uses are also from internal and external uses of herbal extracts.
   a. Analgesic
   b. Antiallergenic
   c. Anti-inflammatory
   d. Antiphlogistic
   e. Antispasmodic
   f. Bactericidal
   g. Carminative
   h. Cicatrizant
   i. Cholagogue
   j. Decongestant
   k. Emmenagogue
   l. Febrifuge
   m. Fungicidal
   n. Hepatic
   o. Nerve sedative
   p. Stimulant of leukocytes
   q. Sudorific
   r. Tonic (digestive and stomachic)
   s. Vermifuge
   t. Vulnerary

6. **Chemical composition:** German chamomile essential oil varies in composition according to the source of harvesting. There are four main chemotypes which have been identified as follows:

♧ **Type A** α-bisabolol oxide Type B > α-bisabolol oxide Type A > α-bisabolol

♧ **Type B** α-bisabolol oxide Type A > α-bisabolol oxide Type B > α-bisabolol

♧ **Type C** α-bisabolol > α-bisabolol oxide Type B > α-bisabolol oxide Type A

♧ **Type D** α-bisabolol oxide Type B = α-bisabolol oxide Type A = α-bisabolol

Battaglia[36]

A typical chemical composition of German chamomile follows: [36]

a. chamazule 2.16% - 35.59%
b. α-bisabolol 1.72% - 76.25%
c. bisabolol oxide, Type A 55.08%
d. bisabolol oxide Type B 4.35 % to 18.93%
e. bisabolone oxide Type A 63.85%

The content and composition of the essential oil are dependent on the development stage of the plant. As an example, the quantity of α-bisabolol, α-bisabolol oxide types A and B, and bisabolone oxide type A reached a maximum in full bloom, whereas the farnesene content decreased rapidly with the growth and development of the flower. [65].

7. **Systems:**

a. Integumentary: Provides support for excessive acne, rosacea, allergies, cuts dermatitis and eczema. Works well with sensitive skin, inflammations, and teething pain. Documented to provide especially good support at a low dose for several leg (skin) ulcers and any damaged skin, especially on severely damaged/infected skin such as cellulitis infections.

b. Muscular/skeletal: Provides support and relief from arthritis, inflamed muscles and joints, neuralgia, and sprains. Can also provide support for rheumatism when combined with yarrow and helichrysum for inflammations

c. Digestive: The herbal extract works well with dyspepsia, colic, indigestion, nausea and gastroduodenal ulcers. May work with the essential oil applied to the affected area of liver regulation and regeneration. Also used as a protective remedy as a tea with rose hydrolat.

d. Genito-urinary/reproductive: Provides support for cystitis, regulates period, and eases pains from PMS and menopausal challenges.

e. Central nervous system: Works well with headaches, insomnia, nervous tension, migraines, and general support for stressful conditions. Possible with internal use, more likely with Roman chamomile for challenges.

8. **Personality:** This beautiful deep blue essential oil exemplifies the personalities of fathers that tuck you in at night, the teacher who helped you with a difficult project, telling you not to worry, and the police officer who accompanied you home when you were in distress. German chamomile personality is kind and caring even to strangers. German chamomile personalities have emotional depth and the ability to draw out of the best in other people but keep their own feelings to themselves, preferring to use a metaphor to disguise how they feel. The character of German chamomile is strong, peaceful, healing, and cooling. These essential oils can be used to encourage positive attributes: communication, relaxation, understanding, organization, soothing, empathy, patience, and calm. This essential oil can be used to counteract these negative attributes: nervousness, frayed nerves, anger, frustration, emotional drama, emotional tension, temper, sensitivity, moodiness, bitterness, resentment, indifference, and deep emotional baggage [66].

9. **Safety:** Reported to be non-toxic, non-irritant, and non-sensitizing.

10. **Blending:** Top/middle.

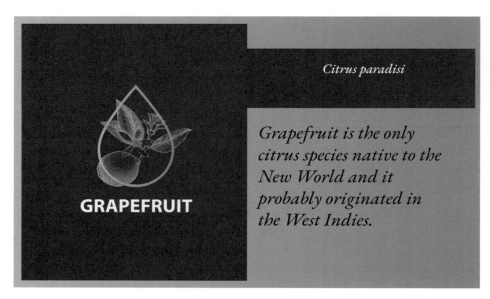

Citrus paradisi

Grapefruit is the only citrus species native to the New World and it probably originated in the West Indies.

Grapefruit
Citrus paradisi

C. paradisi is considered between a hybrid between *C. maxima* and *C. sinensis*. This essential oil is produced in the USA, the West Indies, Brazil, Israel, and Nigeria. The beautiful large fruit is grown on a vigorous tree that grows up to 30m with a single trunk, many branches, and has a round to blunt conical shape if left unpruned. The difference between white and red grapefruit is the generally has a higher aldehyde content in white grapefruit and lower evaporative residue than the red grapefruit, which also contains a small percentage of linalool. Studies indicate that grapefruit oil has considerable antimicrobial activity when tested again *Candida albicans*, *aspergillus niger* and the generally difficult to inhibit *Pseudomonas aeruginosa* [67].

Although *Citrus paradisi* is a circulatory stimulant, the British National Formulary states that anyone taking calcium channel blockers should avoid eating grapefruit or drinking grapefruit juice. In this instance, avoiding the essential oil is highly recommended [68].

Grapefruit may contain up to 98% limonene. Grapefruit oil receives its olfactory character almost entirely from powerful trace components, one of which is the commercial isolated sesquiterpene nootkatone. Its pleasantly refreshing fragrance and rather affordable price makes it very useful for use in diffusers for disinfection of the room air [69].

1. **Class**: Terpenes

2. **Family**: *Rutaceae*

3. **Distillation**: Grapefruit essential oil is expressed from the outside peel of the grapefruit.

4. **Biochemical**:
   a. Monoterpenes: d-limonene (Up to 95%)
   b. Aldehydes: (>2%): nonanal, decanal, citrals, citronellal, and others
   c. Coumarins and furocoumarins: aesculetin, auraptene, limetin, meranzin, bergaptol
   d. Nootkatone (small % but very important in aroma, used to determine harvest time.)

5. **Uses**:
   a. Antiseptic (especially airborne)
   b. Antitoxic
   c. Astringent
   d. Bactericidal
   e. Depurative
   f. Diuretic
   g. Digestive
   h. Lymphatic
   i. Tonic (general)
   j. Stimulant

6. **Chemical composition**: A typical chemical composition of grapefruit essential oil is reported as follows: [67]
   a. α-pinene 0.38%
   b. β--pinene 0.02%
   c. sabinene 0.42%
   d. myrcene 1.37%
   e. d-limonene 84.0%
   f. citronella 0.1%
   g. decanol 0.4%
   h. linalool 0.1%
   i. nootkatone 0.1%

7. **Systems**:
   a. Integumentary: Provides excellent support for athletes' foot, acnes, oily skin, tones and congested skin. Tightens skin, stimulates hair growth, and potentially reduces the appearance of cellulite.
   b. Respiratory: Serves as an airborne disinfectant when diffused.
   c. Muscular/skeletal: Eases muscle fatigue, stiffness.
   d. Cardiovascular: Increases circulation and stimulates lymphatic system detoxification.
   e. Immune: Providers support for cold, chills, and flu. Serves as an excellent environmental disinfectant.
   f. Digestive: Taken internally, stimulates gall bladder and serves as a digestive aid. May be useful in treating anorexia/bulimia. May also provide support as a liver tonic.
   g. Genito-urinary/reproductive: Increases urine flow and eases water retention.
   h. Central nervous system: May provide support for depression, headache, nervous exhaustion, and performance stress. May also provide relief from jet lag, PMS, and alcohol and drug withdrawal. Provides euphoric emotional support, relieving self-doubt and boosting confidence.

8. **Personality**: The grapefruit personality is all about freshness and newness. These are happy, warm people who are usually bursting with energy (even when they are sitting down). They radiate pure energy that gives light to everything they do. Grapefruit personalities love people and they dislike seeing someone who is not fulfilling their potential. They become great motivators, the "get up and go" people, although not overbearing, not saying "do something worthwhile in your life!", rather they give out subtle discreet suggestions, intended to give the recipient confidence or motivation. Their character is

radiating, cheering, joyful, liberating, and boosting. This essential oil encourages positive attributes: joyfulness, positivity, confidence, clarity, balance, inspiration, generosity, uplifted, spontaneity, and cooperation. Grapefruit oil will counteract negative attributes: depression, sadness, grief, apathy, mental pressure, mental exhaustion, emotional violence, self-doubt, self-critics, aggravation, and frustration [70].

9. **Safety**: Caution: grapefruit essential oil is photosensitizing, and the quality of commercially available oils is often dubious. For consistent results, only organic oils should be used [71]. According to Shirley and Len Price, grapefruit oil is non-irritating, non-sensitizing and non-toxic to humans. The aldehydes present make grapefruit essence prone to oxidation; it deteriorates upon expose to moisture, air, and light. The addition of antioxidants is not uncommon as this prolongs the shelf-life, they are effective in concentrations as low as 0.002 percent, which is far below the odor perception threshold [72]. However, care should be taken with external use of expressed grapefruit oil because of possible photosensitization [73].

    According to Sylla Shepphard-Hanger, when tested at low dose, grapefruit essential oil is non-toxic, non-irritant, and non-sensitizing. Odor oxidized oils or those with high d-limonene increases potential for sensitizing. It does appear non-phototoxic [74].

10. **Blending**: Top note.

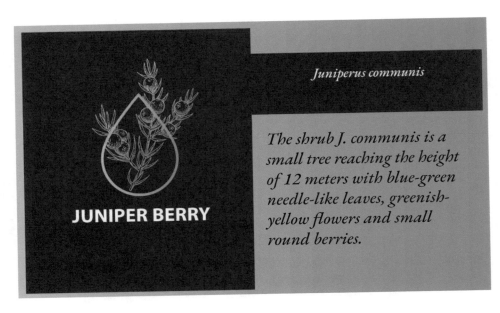

Juniperus communis

The shrub J. communis is a small tree reaching the height of 12 meters with blue-green needle-like leaves, greenish-yellow flowers and small round berries.

Juniper Berry
Juniperus communis

The berries grow wild throughout central Europ andtake about 3 years to mature. According to Battaglia, juniper was commonly burnt as a fumigant and ritual incense by ancient Greeks to combat epidemics, and by Tibetans and native Americans for ceremonial purposes. The German Commission E. Monographs recommends a daily dosage of between 2 and 10 grams of the dried berries for dyspepsia. However, they also warn that prolonged use may cause kidney damage and that it is contraindicated during pregnancy [75].

There is a difference between juniper and juniper berry essential oils. Juniper berry essential oil is produced from the actual fruit. The juniper essential oil is usually redistilled from fermented branches as a by-product of gin manufacturing.

The best quality juniper berries are harvested from northern Italy, Austria, Czech Republic, Hungary, Croatia, Serbia, and France.

1. **Class:** sesquiterpene, monoterpene

2. **Family:** *Cupressaceae*

3. **Distillation:** There are two types of distillations used to produce juniper essential oils: steam distillation and CO_2 extraction.

4. **Biochemical**:
    a. Monoterpenes (mainly): α-pinene (>37%), sabinene, myrcene, limonene, cymene, camphene, γ-terpinene
    b. Sesquiterpene: α-muurolene, cadinene, cedrene
    c. Alcohol: linalool, terpine-4-ol
    d. Aldehydes: camphor, pinocamphone, junionone, thujone
    e. Esters: may include bornyl acetate, terpinyl acetate, coumarins such as umbelliferone

During CO_2 extraction, additional occurring compounds may include:

  ❀ pinenes, terpinene-4-ol, borneol, bornyl and terpinyl acetate (no resins).

5. **Uses**:
    a. Antiseptic (urinary)
    b. Astringent
    c. Anti-infectious
    d. Bactericide (airborne contaminants, staph, strep, pyogenes)
    e. Antidiabetic
    f. Antiarthritic
    g. Antirheumatic
    h. Antispasmodic
    i. Arminative
    j. Cicatrizant
    k. Depurative
    l. Detoxicant
    m. General energy stimulant
    n. Rubefacient
    o. Stimulant (circulatory, respiratory)
    p. Stomachic
    q. Excretory (kidney)
    r. Bladder (diuretic)
    s. Digestive (pancreatic)
    t. Sudorific

u.   Tonic (cardiac)

v.   Vulnerary (wounds)

Notes:

🍂 At low dose, Juniper Berry, stimulates and tones digestive system

🍂 At high dose, it provokes perspiration

🍂 Modified mucus and excretory secretions (especially urine)

6.   **Chemical Composition:** A typical chemical composition of juniper berry is reported as follows: [75]

a.   α-pinene 33.7%

b.   camphene 0.5%

c.   β-pinene 1.1%

d.   sabinene 27.6%

e.   myrcene 5.5%

f.   α-phellandrene 1.3%

g.   α-terpinene 1.9%

h.   y-terpinene 3.0%

i.   1,4-cineol 4%

j.   β-phellandrene 1.3%

k.   para-cymene 5.5%

l.   terpinene-4-ol 4.0%

m.   bornyl acetate 0.4%

n.   caryophyllene 0.6%

o.   traces amount of limonene, camphor, linalool, linalyl acetate, borneol and nerol.

7.   **Systems:**

a.   Integumentary: Provides excellent support for acne, dermatitis, hair loss, and oily skin, especially blocked pores. Works well to relieve varicose veins and cellulite. May aid with eczema, ulcers, abscesses, and edema including simple water retention. Proves support for inflammation, dermatosis, and wounds. Caution: use only low levels with highly diluted oils) on sensitive or damaged skin.

b. Respiratory: Provides support for chronic coryza (head cold) and rhinitis (chronic and intermittent nasal symptoms). Also serves as an excellent airborne disinfectant.

c. Muscular/skeletal: Provides relief from gout pain and rheumatism, especially effective in combination with grapefruit essential oil.

d. Cardiovascular/lymphatic: Provides support for hemorrhoids. Serves as a heart tonic, circulatory stimulant, cleans blood and reduces accumulation of toxins, especially uric acid.

e. Immune: Support for colds, flu, and infections

f. Digestive: May help with toothache pain. Supports detox from overindulgence in food and alcohol. Stimulates pancreatic digestion, eases gout, supports intestinal colitis caused by infections.

g. Genito-urinary/reproductive: Eases menstruation pain. Provides support for leucorrhea, cystitis, and genital warts. Stimulates kidney and bladder

h. Central nervous system: Provides support for anxiety, nervous tension, stress related challenges, jet lag, poor memory, and overall weakness. Strengthens and uplifts mood and Emotions. Clears negative energy from room (especially before meditation). Facilitates love and positive mental energy.

8. **Personality**: The juniper personality can be radical in their lack of concern for human authority, professing to be directed by intuition or religious belief. They have a reverence for anything sacred and will inevitably take a spiritual path through life, although the form of spirituality varies greatly. The juniper personality doesn't consciously seek out spiritual places but seems to be drawn to them. The character of juniper personality is cleaning, purifying, sacred, and visionary. This oil encourages positive attributes of self-worth, spirituality,

peace, inner vision, strength, vitality, cleansing, meditation, conviction, enlightenment, wisdom, and humility. This essential oil counteracts these negative attributes: nervous exhaustion, emotional exhaustion, guilt, lack of self-worth, dissatisfaction, anxiety, abuse, transience, emptiness, conflict, and defensiveness [76].

9. **Safety**: Tested at low dosages, general non-toxic, non-sensitizing, rubefacient effect, so avoid extensive use on delicate skin. Avoid in kidney disease, acute kidney-bladder infections. Avoid in pregnancy. This essential oil has a strong diuretic effect and prolonged use can damage kidneys. According to Battaglia, he agrees with Tisserand and Balac, who state there is a good chance that juniper oil may be confused with savin, whose botanical name is *J. sabina* [77].

10. **Blending**: Middle note.

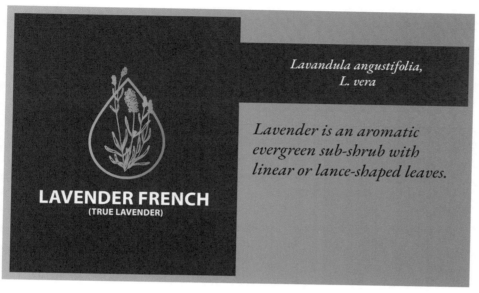

Lavandula angustifolia, L. vera

Lavender is an aromatic evergreen sub-shrub with linear or lance-shaped leaves.

Lavender French (True Lavender)
Lavandula angustifolia, L. vera

It grows up to 0.9 m high and is native to the Mediterranean region. The lavandula genus has approximately 30 species that grow around the world and the four main species of lavender include:

- *L. angustifolia* - True lavender
- *L. latifolia* - Spike lavender
- *L. x intermedia* - Lavandin
- *L. stoechas* - Maritime lavender

The main producers of true lavender are Bulgaria and France. Smaller producers include Australia, Argentina, England, Hungary, Japan, Morocco, Italy, Algeria, India, and Russia. Chapter 2, Lesson 9 provides additional information on lavender essential oils.

Lavender is one of the most commonly adulterated essential oils. Adulteration of true lavender in the essential oil trade is common and often includes [78]:

- Addition of lavandin essential oil
- Substitution of lavandin essential oil
- Addition of synthetic linalool and linalyl acetate
- Addition of linalool and linalyl acetate from other sources.

According to Scott Johnson, some reports suggest lavender contains significant amounts of 1,8 cineol (eucalyptol); however, these may be misidentified lavandin or spike lavender (*Lavandula spica*) samples, or adulterated samples. Lavender essential oil is often adulterated with lavandin. Shorter distillation times also increase the 1,8-cineol content of lavender essential oils. [79]

Marcel Lavabre references lavender as one of the most precious essential oils. Lavender was a favorite aromatic used by the Romans in their baths. Dioscorides, Pliny, and Galen mention it as a stimulant, tonic, stomachic and carminative. It has always been used in perfumery and cosmetics and combines easily with many essential oils, adding a light, floral note to almost any preparation. The finest quality grows above 3,000 feet on the sunny slopes of the southern Alps and up to the mountain tops. [80]

Approximately half of the true lavender is produced using cultivated clones such as maillette (*Lavandula angustifolia*). Maillette is a selection of lavender grown both in France and England for the high yield and quality of its sweet-smelling oil. The flowerheads of maillette are packed full of tiny plum to lilac star-shaped flowers and are barrel-shaped rather than spiked. This gives a 40 to 50 percent higher yield than population lavender (meaning raised from seed.) D.R. Harris says that popular lavender from France has a superior fragrance and commands a higher price than cloned lavender and lavender from other countries. [81] Lavandulol and its ester lavandulyl acetate contribute to the aroma of this oil [82], known as "true" lavender. Sylla Sheppard-Hanger suggests that L. *spica* is suitable for making lavender wands and baskets because of the long-stemmed flowers [83] However, the scent can be rather harsh.

1. **Class**: Ester, alcohol

2. **Family**: *Lamiaceae* (*Labiatae*)

3. **Distillation**: Steam distillation from the flowers and stalks.

4. **Biochemical**: According to Sylla-Sheppard-Hangar, this lavender is the most commercially traded lavender and is harvested from various growing regions, sub-varieties, clones.

   It is often mixed or blended, so tremendous chemical variation occurs in the final products. Cloning has also produced more vigorous hybrids. Growers may have to go back to wilder varieties for increased resistance referring to the hardiness of the plant as well as the effectiveness of the oil produced. Constituents vary with growing conditions and locations. (i.e., - linalool acetate alone varies from 9.08% to 54%. From plants grown in high altitudes, the oil produces more esters.

a. Monoterpenes: (>5): α-pinene, camphene, 3-carene, cis & trans-ocimenes, allo-ocimene, limonene
b. Sesquiterpenes: β-caryophyllene, β-farnesene
c. Alcohols: linalool (>41%), smaller amounts of terpinen-4-ol, α-terpineol, borneol, geraniol, lavandulol, nerol
d. Esters (approx. 50%): linalyl acetate, terpenyl acetate, geranyl, and lavandulyl acetate
e. Oxides: 1,8 cineol, linaloxide, caryophyllene oxide
f. Ketones: camphor
g. Also: aldehydes, lactones, coumarins, and other of low molecular weight: octanol-3, octanone-3, hexyl butyrate, acetocy-3-octene-1

The Tasmania lavender also includes linalool, and linalyl acetate. The Yugoslavian lavender contains linalool, camphor, and limonene.

5. Uses:
    a. Analgesic
    b. Anticonvulsive
    c. Antidepressant
    d. Antimicrobial
    e. Anti-infectious
    f. Antiphlogistic
    g. Antirheumatic
    h. Antiseptic
    i. Antispasmodic
    j. Antitoxic
    k. Antiviral
    l. Bactericide

m.   Carminative
n.   Cholagogue
o.   Cicatrizant
p.   Choleretic
q.   Cordial
r.   Cytophylactic
s.   Decongestant
t.   Deodorant
u.   Diuretic
v.   Emmenagogue
w.   Fungicide
x.   Hypotensive
y.   Insecticide
z.   Nervine
aa. Parasiticide
ab. Restorative
ac. Rubefacient
ad. Sedative
ae. Stimulant
af. Sudorific
ag. Tonic (general neurotonic, cardiac regulator)
ah. Vasodilator
ai. Vulnerary

6.   **Chemical composition**: A typical chemical composition of lavender is [84]:
   a. α-pinene – 0.02 - 0.67%
   b.   limonene – 0.02 - 0.68%
   c.   1,8 cineol 0.01 - 0.21%
   d.   cis-ocimene – 1.35 - 2.87%
   e.   trans-ocimene – 0.86 - 1.36%
   f.   3-octanone – 1.75 - 3.04%
   g.   camphor – 0.54 - 0.89%
   h.   linalool – 29.35 - 41.62%
   i.   linalyl acetate – 46.71 - 53.80%
   j.   caryophyllene – 2.64 - 5.05%
   k.   terpinen-4-ol – 0.03 - 4.16%
   l.   lavandulyl acetate – 0.27 - 4.24%

The chart below was compiled from the book "Evidence Based Essential Oil Therapy" by Dr. Scott A Johnson. Several constituents occurring in lower percentages are not included in this table. The Brazilian oil includes five other different compounds not listed here. The English oil contains three other compounds not listed, and the Munstead (UK) essential oil contains one other compound not listed. However, this table demonstrates the difference in chemical composition of oils from worldwide sources. [85]

	English	Munstead	Brazilian	Bulgarian	French	Indian	Italian	Polish
linalool	24.5-50.6%	37.8-46.1%		25.4-47.3%	9.3-68.8%	26.7-37.1%	33.3-45.0%	27.3-34.7%
linalyl acetate	3.7 - 45.0%	6.1 - 12.2%		19.9-37.6%	1.2-59.4%	35.4-49.5%	31.7%-41.2%	19.7%-22.4%
caryophyllene	0.0 - 24.!							
1,8 cineol	0.0 - 19.8%		7.9%	0.4-4.2%	0.0-3.4%			
β-phellandrene	0.0-16.0%							
sabinene	0.1-11.0%							
terpinen-4-ol	7.8-9.6%	0.3-19.5%		0.1-7.4%	0.1-13.5%		1.1-3.6%	1.1-2.0%
(z)- β-ocimene	0.0-7.8%			1.7-7.7%				
lavandulyl acetate	2.7-6.4%			2.5-4.4%	0.3-21.6%	0.6-4.5%		4.5-5.7%
β-caryophyllene	2.0-6.1%			1.7-5.2%		0.9-4.0%		
α-terpineol	1.5-6.0%	19.2-20.6%				1.2-3.8%		
borneol	0.4-5.1%		22.4%					
ocimene					0.2-18.1%			1.9-2.9%
cymene		4.8-8.3%						
lavandulol					0.0-4.3%			
ocimene								1.9-2.0%
germacrene d	0.2-4.7%							
trans- β-ocimene				1.0-4.2%				

7. Systems:

   a. Integumentary: Supports all skin types especially dry and/or oily skin by balancing the sebum. Excellent support for eczema, psoriasis, pruritus, bruises, and burns, especially sunburns. Provides healing for scars and thread veins. Aids wound healing, abscesses, ulcers, and soothes skin pain, especially health challenges that involve splitting of dermis and epidermis by soothing pain and regenerating cells.

b. Respiratory: Provides support for bronchitis, catarrh, colds, and laryngitis. May support asthma and other respiratory pathologies of the nervous origin. Relaxes and eases breathing.

c. Muscular/skeletal: Support for muscle spasms, sprains, strains, cramps, and muscular contracture. Provides relief for rheumatic pain and chronic rheumatism.

d. Cardiovascular/lymphatic: Lowers or balances high blood pressure. Serves as an anticoagulant (blood thinner) and eases heart palpitations. Potential support for retinal periphlebitis. Provides support during arteritis and coronaritis. Supports circulatory deficiency by increasing capillary circulation. Supports lymphatic detoxification.

e. Immune: Supports flu, viral infections, typhus, and tuberculosis.

f. Digestive: Provides supports for teething pain, clears spleen and liver, increases liver circulation, stimulates bile production, and aids with nausea, vomiting and colic. Promotes digestion and eases solar plexus spasm.

g. Genito-urinary/reproductive: Provides relief during childbirth pain and hastens delivery. May aid with scanty periods, cystitis, and thrush.

h. Central nervous system: Works with brain and central nervous system as a sedative. May also support headaches, nervous tension, and exhaustion. Provides support for manic depression, mood swings, and anger.

8. **Personality**: Lavender could be called the mother or grandmother of essential oil, able to care for a multitude of physical and psychological problems. Similar to a mother's responsibility, this personality can accomplish several jobs at the same time. Even in times of hardship, the lavender personality bravely continues overcoming obstacles that are placed in their way. The character of a lavender is consistently harmonious, calming, healing, caring, compassionate and embracing. Lavender encourages positive attributes including security, gentleness, reconciliation, clarity, comfort, acceptance, inner peace, relaxation, alertness, emotionally balanced, visualization, and rejuvenation. Lavender will counteract these negative attributes: anxiety, stress, tension, mental exhaustion, panic, apprehension, nightmares, insecurity, loss of inner child, obsessional behavior, trauma, jitteriness, depression, psychosomatic illness, nervousness, worry, over-excitedness, and burnout. [86].

9. **Safety**: Tested at low dose, non-toxic, non-irritant, non-sensitizing; rare photosensitization reported. Permitted to be used as food flavor. non-hazardous in pregnancy.

10. **Blending**: Top/middle note.

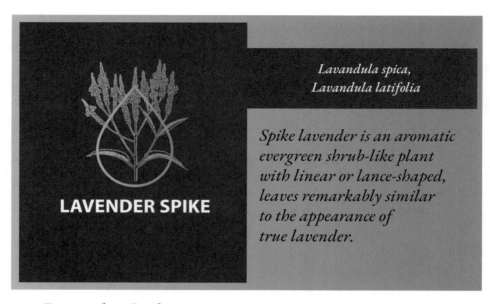

Lavandula spica,
Lavandula latifolia

Spike lavender is an aromatic evergreen shrub-like plant with linear or lance-shaped, leaves remarkably similar to the appearance of true lavender.

Lavender Spike
Lavandula spica, Lavandula latifolia

It is easily distinguished from other lavender species by long, spatula-shaped leaves and long flowering spikes with grayish-blue flowers. This aromatic plant grows wild around the Mediterranean countries, particularly Spain, France and Italy. Spain is the major producer of the oil. Commonly called aspic, it is considered to be "male lavender" in contrast to *L. angustifolia*, which is referred to as "female lavender."

Nicholas Culpeper (1616-1654) was one of the most influential herbalists who also introduced the concept of astrological herbalism. In "*The English Physician*" (1652), he was one of the first to translate from Latin documents discussing medicinal plants found in the Americas. His herbal expertise was held in such esteem that species he described were introduced into the New World (Americas) from England. Culpeper described the medical use of the foxglove, the botanical precursor to digitalis, to treat heart conditions.

Culpeper's descriptions of herbs, oils and their uses recommended spike lavender for a variety of ailments such as pains in the head and brain, falling sickness, dropsy, cramps, and convulsions. He described the oil of spike lavender as having a fierce and piercing quality, and recommended using the oil cautiously, a few drops being sufficient for inward and outward griefs [87].

Kurt Schnaubelt suggests that experience and research demonstrates essential oils that contain either strongly electrophilic (phenols or terpenes alcohols) or strongly nucleophilic (citral) constituents are most effective treating diseases caused by hulled viruses. Particular effectiveness has been found with essential oils with a built-in-energy of terpene alcohols and cineol [88]

Essential oils	Synergy
♣ *Ravensara aromatica* ♣ *Laurus nobilis* ♣ *Eucalyptus radiata* ♣ *Melaleuca viridiflora* (Niaouli)	♣ α-terpineol/cineole
♣ *Melaleuca alternifolia* ♣ *Melaleuca linariifolia*	♣ terpineol-4-cineol
♣ *Eucalyptus globulous*	♣ pinocarveol/cineol
♣ *Lavandula spica*	♣ linalool/cineol

Viruses are infectious, subcellular particles. They consist of DNA or RNA—genetic material surrounded (in the case of "hulled" viruses) by a protein or lipoprotein "coat". This hull protects the nucleic acid and also provides, in diverse ways, for the virus' ability to invade other cells. Viruses are independent genetic systems that take over the cell's machinery, causing it to synthesize virus protein and virus-nucleic acid and, according to the blueprint, synthesizes the enveloped proteins. Their replication within the living cell and transfer through infection cause characteristic reactions in the host cell and in the host organisms [89]. Therefore, the above-mentioned aromatic medicine which may support elimination of the viruses from the cell is important to know which synergy they have within the constituents.

1. **Class:** Alcohol, ketone, oxide

2. **Family:** *Labiatae* or *Lamiaceae*

3. **Distillation:** Spike lavender is steam distilled from the flowering tops of *L. spica*. Most spike lavender is distilled from wild plants.

4. **Biochemical:**
   a. Monoterpenes (>10%) α- & β-pinene, camphene, limonene
   b. Sesquiterpenes: (>3%) β-caryophyllene, β-bisabolene
   c. Alcohols: linalool, terpinen-4-ol, α-terpineol, smaller amounts of terpinen-4-ol, α terpineol, borneol, geraniol, citronellol, lavandulol, nerol, octenol-3.
   d. Esters: (>2%) linalyl acetate,
   e. Oxides: (<35%) 1,8 cineol (>39%), caryophyllene oxide, trans & cis-linalool oxide
   f. Coumarins: coumarin, herniarin

5. **Uses:**
   a. Analgesic
   b. Antidepressant
   c. Antiseptic
   d. Anti-infectious
   e. Antimycosis (coli bacillus, staph, intestinal)
   f. Anti-inflammatory
   g. Bactericidal (staph)
   h. Antiviral
   i. Cytophylactic
   j. Emmenagogue (light)
   k. Fungicide
   l. Immunostimulant
   m. Decongestant
   n. Expectorant
   o. Insecticide
   p. Tonic (general cardiac)
   q. Veterinary use: external with turpentine using minute dilutions: rheumatism, hoof problems, cuts, bruises, scabies, eczema, after exercising animals, dog arthritis, synovial dilations, traumas; digestive problems, and tonic.

6. **Chemical composition:** The main difference between spike lavender and true lavender is the high camphor and

1,8 cineol content of spike lavender. The description of French or true lavender for comparisons is provided above. A typical composition of spike lavender is: [84]

    a.   α-pinene   1.7%
    b.   camphene   0.5%
    c.   β-pinene   1.5%
    d.   myrcene   1.4%
    e.   1,8 cineole   23.5%
    f.   para-cymene   0.6%
    g.   camphor   20.0%
    h.   linalool   32.4%
    i.   terpinen-4-ol   1.5%
    j.   borneol   4.6%
    k.   geraniol   1.8%

7.   **Systems**:

    a.   Integumentary: Provides support for severe burns, dry acne, fungal infections, and athletes' foot (with *orania mixta*, a species of sea snail, a marine gastropod mollusk in the family Muricidae, the murex snails or rock snails), insect stings, insect bites, scar tissue formation, ringworm, wound healing, antiseptic, abscesses (to facilitate the infection coming to a head), scars, and ulcers.

    b.   Respiratory: Provides support for bronchitis, laryngitis, rhinitis, sore throat, coughs, must be used with rosemary cineole for any respiratory cough, tonsilitis, (strep and β-hemolytic with thyme linalool) and ear infections.

    c.   Muscular/skeletal: Support for rheumatic pain (with rosemary cineole, ravensara), muscle pain, paralysis, and rheumatoid arthritis.

    d.   Cardiovascular: As a mild cardiotonic, increases blood pressure.

    e.   Immune: Provides support for flu and viral infections. Serves as an immuno-stimulant (equal strength of chemical constituent alcohols) and is well suited for children above the age of 12.

    f.   Digestive: Provides relief of flatulence, dyspepsia, colic, and colitis (viral). Eases teething pain (application of diluted oil during a jaw massage).

    g.   Genito-urinary/reproductive: Induces menstruation (light) and regulates and eases cramps when used with sage blend.

    h.   Central nervous system: Provides support for asthenia, neuritis, neuralgia, debility, and depressive headache. Aids headache pain, neuritis (when used with peppermint) and serves as a cerebral-spinal tranquilizer. Calms senses, cleansing and balancing.

8.   **Personality**: This is definitely a male oil defined as "Yang." Picking *Lavandula spica* is a pleasant experience, certainly less "heady" than with Lavandula vera, but nevertheless, profound due to its closeness to nature in the wild [90]. *Lavandula spica* personality is someone characteristic of our time, searching for sound values and a new awareness —though well anchored in today's world, he wants to materialize his dreams of tomorrow out of sync with the world as he is with himself, but this is undoubtedly part of his own equilibrium and his picturesque charm. Physically, this character tends to focus less on appearance and may resemble a student from the 1960s who has come down from his barricades to go and climb hills: long-haired, bearded, and disheveled, even scruffy in appearance. The lavender personality is staunch and very intelligent. Of a kindly, albeit sometimes shady nature, this personality can also be asocial and retreat into an entropic life, living off the land including goat's milk and farm eggs [91].

9.   **Safety**: The camphor content varies between 10 to 20 percent and the 1,8-cineol content varies between 25 and 35 percent. As camphor is considered a neurotoxic,

it is possible spike lavender may be neurotoxic as well. Robert Tisserand also suggests that it would only be contraindicated when taken orally. [92] Do not take with preparations containing iodine or iron [93]. Avoid any use during pregnancy.

10. **Blending**: Top note.

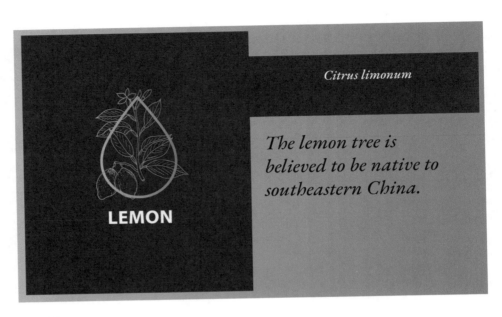

Citrus limonum

LEMON

The lemon tree is believed to be native to southeastern China.

Lemon
Citrus limonum

Arriving in Europe via Persia and the Middle East with returning soldiers from religious crusades in the 12th century [94]. Lemon fruit trees grow year-round with the deep green fruits that ripen to a bright yellow color. Lemon essential oil is mostly cultivated from trees in California, Florida, and southern Europe.

Lemon juice has been used as a restorative throughout history, including its effectiveness as a remedy for scurvy (scorbutic). English ships were required by law to carry sufficient lemon or lime juice for every seaman to ingest once daily after being at sea for ten days or more [95]. Lemon oil is extensively used in pharmaceuticals as a flavoring agent and as a fragrance ingrediency in commercially produced soaps, detergents, and perfumes.

Lemon oil exhibits antimicrobial properties. Studies in Japan found that when dispersed through the room, lemon oil reduced typing errors by 54 percent [96].

Kurt Schnaubelt surmises that in the last several years, lemon essential oil has received renewed public interest through the discovery of the antitumor effects of limonene. For use in aromatherapy, lemon oil should be obtained exclusively from organically grown fruits that are pesticide free, because industrially cultivated citrus plantations are invariably sprayed with heavy doses of toxic chemicals. Lemon essential oil has strong anti-infectious and antiviral activity and can be an effective component of blends aimed at liver regeneration and detoxification. Recently, a range of influences of limonene on receptor-mediated processes have been documented showing antiviral activity used as a component of blends aimed at liver regeneration and detoxification and showing it to be preventative and curative for breast cancer in early studies. Lemon essential oil strengthens capillaries by diminishing their permeability. His recommended application is short-term only, either internally or topically. In order to achieve aromatherapy and healing, the essential oil must be unadulterated, obtained through organic production and harvest. [97]

According to the research by Dr. Scott Johnson [98], inhaling lavender, lemon and ylang-ylang oils (2:2:1 ratio) reduced systolic blood pressure and influenced heart rate and sympathetic nervous system activity in people with essential hypertension (also called primary hypertension; high blood pressure without identifiable cause). Inhalation of lemon oil balances the autonomic nervous system (ANS) as an adaptogen. The impact on ANS activity differed greatly between healthy and depressed patients. Healthy subjects experienced increased sympathetic and parasympathetic activity after inhalation, whereas depressed persons experienced increased parasympathetic activity. Sympathetic nervous system activity is often elevated, and parasympathetic activity decreased in people who are depressed [99].

The anticoagulant property of lemon oil is described in energetic terms as an ability to "move the blood," a therapeutic effect that depends partly on its astringent nature. Improving circulation and toning the blood vessels, lemon essential oil may support healing for broken capillaries, varicose veins, hemorrhoids, and nosebleeds. [100]

According to Sylla Sheppard-Hanger, lemon essential oil can also be produced through rectification of the "bergapten-free or "green" lemon. Despite the name, the fruit varies from yellow to orange, depending on its color when picked. While lemon essential oil is considered antiseptic when freshly distilled, essential oils can lose this specific characteristic within weeks as it ages. Most commercially traded oils are several months old by the time they are sold; therefore, the chemical characteristic is no longer effective. Lemon juice is much stronger than the lemon essential oil, and as a cancer preventative, the juice may produce more favorable activity than the essential oils. [101]

1.   **Class**: Monoterpene

2.   **Family**: *Rutaceae*

3. **Distillation**: Distilled using the cold expression method.

4. **Biochemical:**
   a. Monoterpenes: d-limonene (highest up to 72%), α-& y-terpinene, paracymene, α-& β-phellandrene, terpinolene, terpinene, pinene, sabinene
   b. Sesquiterpenes: β-bisabolene
   c. Alcohols: hexanol, octanol, nonanol, decanol, 3-hexene-1-ol, n-heptanol, linalool, geraniol
   d. Aldehydes (>3%): hexanol, heptanal, octanal, nonanal, geranial, neral
   e. Coumarins & furocoumarins (>5%): scopoletine, umbelliferone, trans-r-bergamotene, bergaptol, bergaptene, citroptene, 8-geranoxy-psoralen, 5-geranoxy, 8-methoxypsoralene

5. **Uses:**
   a. Adaptogen
   b. Antianemic
   c. Antibacterial (strep, spore bacteria)
   d. Antifungal
   e. Antimicrobial
   f. Antirheumatic
   g. Antitoxic
   h. Antisclerotic
   i. Antiscorbutic
   j. Antiseptic (fresh lemon juice)
   k. Antispasmodic
   l. Astringent
   m. Bactericidal
   n. Carminative
   o. Cicatrizant
   p. Depurative
   q. Diaphoretic
   r. Diuretic
   s. Febrifuge
   t. Hemostatic
   u. Hypotensive

v.   Insecticidal
w.   Rubefacient
x.   Stimulates white corpuscles
y.   Tomachic
z.   Tonic (calming nerves, digestion)
aa. Vermifuge
ab. Vasoconstrictor

6. **Chemical composition:** Lemon essential oil is comprised mostly of limonene (up to 70%), a monoterpene hydrocarbon. A typical chemical composition of lemon is reported as follows: [77]

   a.   α-pinene – 18. - 3.6%
   b.   camphene – 0.0 - 0.1%
   c.   β-pinene – 6.1 - 15.0%
   d.   sabinene – 1.5 - 4.6%
   e.   myrcene – 1.0 - 2.1%
   f.   α-terpinene – 0.0 - 0.5%
   g.   linalool – 0.0 - 0.9%
   h.   β-bisabolene – 0.0 - 0.56%
   i.   limonene – 62.1 - 74.5%
   j.   trans- α-bergamotene – 0.37%
   k.   nerol – 0.04%
   l.   neral – 0.76%

7. **Systems**:

   a.   Integumentary: Provides support for mouth ulcers, herpes, acne, boils, corns, warts, thin hair, and nails. Improves shine of hair and stimulates hair growth. Strengthen epidermis function and aids epidermal circulation including gland stimulation and purification. Tightens blood vessels. Stimulates connective tissue elastin and collagen. May protect against infection, aid in the development of acid mantle, and lightens skin pigments.

   b.   Respiratory: Provides support for asthma, sore throat, bronchitis, catarrhal, sinus infections, and all respiratory infections. To address respiratory challenges, diffusion and inhalation are the most effective applications.

c. Muscular/skeletal: Provides support for arthritis, tightens and smooths muscles, and strengthens connective tissue.

d. Cardiovascular: Provides effective support for poor circulation and high blood pressure. Provides relief for nose bleeds and tightens smooth muscles of blood vessels. Provides support similar to Vitamin P for capillary circulation. Prevents hypertensive or diabetic accidents. Thins blood. Excellent support for phlebitis, varicose veins, thrombosis, and arteriosclerosis.

e. Immune: Provides support for colds, flu, fever, contagious infections, and congestion. Clears airborne bacteria. Excellent for local disinfection. Stimulates white blood cells and serves as a possible cancer preventative (more likely with use of fresh lemon juice rather than the essential oil).

f. Digestive: Provides support for dyspepsia, constipation, detoxification, and obesity. Outstanding liver cleanser and pancreatic stimulant for insulin. Reduces blood sugar, counters anemia, and balances stomach acidity. Stimulates gland secretions and alimentary canals to relax and smooth cells including pancreas, gallbladder, and stomach.

g. Endocrine: Acts as a stimulant.

h. Genito-urinary/reproductive: Induces labor when overdue, by stimulating the vasopressin releases causing vasoconstricting effect on kidneys and reduced urine excretion. Aids with nephritic colic, stimulates all gland secretion and relax cells for smooth, efficient reproductive organs (uterus, fallopian tubes). Aids with candida infections including thrush.

i. Central nervous system: Serves as stimulant for the brain, all sense organs, and parasympathetic nervous system. Clears thought, aids concentration, and promotes spiritual and psychic awareness. Promotes connection between spirit and mind (consciousness and soul) and is wonderful for use to resolve conflicting thoughts and encourage intellect. Acts as cooling and calming for the CNS.

8. **Personality**: Lemon personality types are lively and casual, unbothered by the struggles and strains of living, able to take it all quite calmly, dealing with each problem as it comes along. A lemon personality's enthusiasm seems to rub off onto people around them, with subtle and permanent effect. As lemons personalities are often workaholics, they are inevitably under stress and when the crunch comes, everyone is in their firing line. Their mood can swing quickly and unexpectedly, confusing those around them, as positivity turns to negative emotions. Thus, the character for lemon can be purifying, stimulating, directional, and versatile. This essential oil encourages these positive attributes: joy, emotional clarity, direction, concentration, liveliness, consciousness, strength, clarity of thought, memory, and emotional invigoration. Lemon essential oil can be used to counteract these negative attributes: resentfulness, depression, bitterness, touchiness, lethargy, humorless, indecisiveness, bad attitudes, distrust, mental blocks, stress, mental fatigue, turmoil, irrationality, and fear [102].

9. **Safety**: According to Scott Johnson, this oil may be photosensitizing when cold-pressed/expressed. Avoid sun exposure to area of application for at least 12 hours after topical application.[103] According to Mojay, lemon essential oil is non-toxic, non-irritant; however, sensitization can occur in some people. Lemon essential

oil should not be used on the skin prior to sun exposure as it is phototoxic. Sunbed rays or direct sunlight should be avoided up to 12 hours following application of the diluted essential oil to the skin [104]. Again, avoid all use on sensitive or damaged skin, as it is phototoxic.

10. **Blending**: Top note.

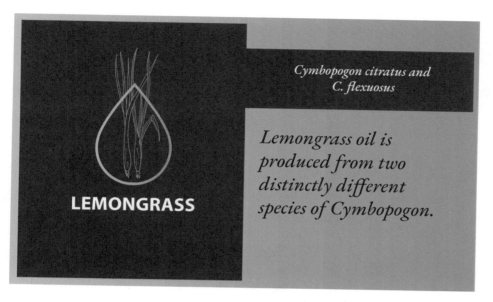

Cymbopogon citratus and
C. flexuosus

Lemongrass oil is
produced from two
distinctly different
species of Cymbopogon.

Lemongrass
Cymbopogon citratus and C. flexuosus

C. *citratus* and C. *flexuosus* are tufted perennial grasses with numerous, stiff stems arising from a short rhizomatous rootstock. C. *flexuosus* is a native of India and C. *citratus* is possibly a native of Sri Lanka. C. *citratus* is widely cultivated all over the world and has been named the West Indian lemongrass [105]. According to the Indian pharmacopeia, lemongrass was traditionally used by the West Indian people as an antidote against infectious diseases, fever, and cholera [106].

A study found that lemongrass essential oil exhibited a significant anticonvulsant effect on mice. The researchers also concluded that the mechanism of action of the anticonvulsant effect of lemongrass is, at least in part, dependent on the gamma-aminobutyric acid (GABA) neurotransmission. Activation of the GABA receptor system and the blockade of neuronal voltage-gate sodium channels are essential for the overall balance between neuronal excitation and inhibition which is vital for normal brain function and critical for the central nervous system disorders. This essential oil constituents may exert their biological activities by modulating the GABA system and inhibiting sodium channels. It was also reported that the effect of lemongrass oil on anti-inflammatory biomarkers can also contribute to their CNS activity [107].

1. **Class**: Aldehyde

2. **Family**: *Gramineae* or *Poaceae*

3. **Distillation**: Steam distilled from fresh or partly dried leaves of *C. citratus* or *C. flexuosus*.

4. **Biochemical**:
    a. Monoterpenes: limonene (>11%), myrcene, dipentene
    b. Aldehydes (>87%): citrals (neral & geranial), citronellal, isovaleric aldehyde, furfural, n-dicyclic aldehyde
    c. Esters: valeric, caprylic, and capric
    d. Alcohols: citronellol, nerol, geraniol, linalool, terpineol, isopulegol and others. Also: methyl-heptenone

5. **Uses**:
    a. Analgesic
    b. Antidepressant
    c. Anti-inflammatory
    d. Antimicrobial (strep and staph pyogenes var. *aureus, e. coli, proteus vulgaris, b. subtilis* [vegetative as spores], *strep faecalis*)
    e. Antioxidant
    f. Antirachitic
    g. Antiseptic (strong airborne)
    h. Astringent
    i. Bactericidal
    j. Carminative
    k. Deodorant
    l. Febrifuge
    m. Fungicidal
    n. Parasiticide
    o. Galactagogue
    p. Insecticidal
    q. Nervine

r.   Sedative (CNS)

s.   Tonic (digestive)

t.   Vasodilator

External veterinary use includes support to prevent parasites and scabies. Internal veterinary internal use includes indigestion and gas.

6.   **Chemical composition**: A typical chemical composition of lemongrass is reported as:

Constituent	*C. flexuosus*	*C. citratus*
myrcene	0.46%	8.2 - 19.2%
limonene	2.42%	trace
linalool	1.34%	0.8 - 1.1%
citronellal	0.37%	0.1%
geranyl acetate	1.95%	1.00%
nerol	0.39%	0.3 - 0.4%
geraniol	3.8%	0.5 - 0.4%
neral	30.06%	25 – 28%
geranial	51.19%	45.2 - 55.9%
citronellol	0.44%	0.1%

C. citratus has a slightly lower citral content and a significant higher amount of myrcene. (Battaglia [107])

7.   **Systems**:

    a.   Integumentary: Provides support for acne, athletes' foot, skin parasites, bruises, excessive perspiration, enlarged pores, oil skin and hair, tissue toner. Stimulates hydration and lymphatic detoxification. Aids weak connective tissue and tightens elastin weakness.

    b.   Muscular/skeletal: Provides support for arthritis and after sport-muscle pain (sprain, bruises, dislocation). Improves muscle tone and is especially good for connective tissue.

   c.   Cardiovascular: May aid with arthritis. Stops bleeding, increases circulation, increases lymphatic circulation, and supports detoxification.

   d.   Immune: Provides support for fevers and infections. Aids environment disinfection. Can also serve as a deodorant. Supports thymus gland and activates resistant cells.

   e.   Digestive: Provides support for colitis, indigestion, and gastroenteritis. Stimulates liver and digestion. Serves as an intestinal antiseptic and fights intestinal parasites.

   f.   Endocrine: Supports thymus gland and spleen function.

   g.   Genito-urinary/reproductive: Induces menstruation and increases milk in nursing mothers.

   h.   Central nervous system: Acts as a sedative. Provides support for headaches and similar stress related conditions. Helps with nervous exhaustion, irritability, lack of concentration, and morning fatigue.

8.   **Personality**: Philippe Mailhebiau, in the book "Portraits in Oils", states that "its powerful, warm odor is an excellent cerebral stimulator and a nerve tonic for those who doubt themselves" [109]. When mixed with Ravensara aromatica, a power nerve tonic, it brings a powerful, exorcising fire, affording the person the opportunity of a certain degree of self-domination. "Lemongrass is a secrete aid for people who have trouble getting started in the morning because it is not only a psychologically refreshing, but also serves as a tonic for tightening weak connective tissue" [110]. "Lemongrass essential oil enables the mind to shift towards fascinating about what is possible, encouraging you to embark on a glorious voyage of discovery. Imagine the circumference of your life experience expanding.

If something has been achieved out of the wide world, then know that it is possible for you to achieve it too." [111] When unable to concentrate or experiencing morning grumpiness, or tiredness from travel, lemongrass is the perfect solution as a refreshing tonic. [112]

9. **Safety**: Lemongrass oil may irritate sensitive skin when used as a compress, or facial oil. Caution is advised during pregnancy and lactation due to the high citral and beta-myrcene content. Large doses of citral may negatively affect fetal development according to animal studies, and extremely high doses of beta-myrcene have been toxic to fetuses in similar research. Use cautiously with diabetic medications. May interact with antibiotics and possibly enhance their effects. There is a moderate risk that when lemongrass is taken orally it may interfere with enzymes responsible for metabolizing medications (NSAIDS, proton pump inhibitors, acetaminophen, antiepileptics, immune modulators, blood sugar medication, blood pressure medications, antihistamines, antibiotics, and anesthetics [Johnson, 150]) According to Robert Tisserand, this essential oil exhibits drug interactions on all routes, teratogenicity, and skin sensitization, especially when taken orally with diabetes medication and pregnancy by being metabolized by CYP2B6 (analgesics, opioids, anesthetics, anticonvulsants, antidepressants, chemotherapeutic drugs, glucocorticoids, nicotine, and reverse-transcriptase inhibitors [114]. Avoid any use during pregnancy.

10. **Blending**: Top note.

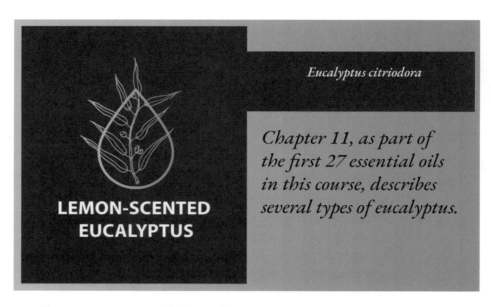

Eucalyptus citriodora

Chapter 11, as part of the first 27 essential oils in this course, describes several types of eucalyptus.

Lemon-scented Eucalyptus
Eucalyptus citriodora

Eucalyptus citriodora is also a worthwhile oil to study and identify healing purposes. As an inexpensive and effective wellness support, *Eucalyptus citriodora* provides anti-inflammative support for arthritis, especially when used in combination with Helichrysum italicum. This oil relieves muscular tensions, and its wonderful sedative qualities are supportive to treat of sleeplessness. *Eucalyptus citriodora* is often preferred over citronella since it has become available in organic quality from produced in east Africa. Dr. Schnaubelt's preferred mode of use is external only and the quality is available in nonindustrial and organic (Medical Aromatherapy, 200).

Lemon-scented eucalyptus is a medium to tall tree up to 50 meters in height with a single stem. Most of the trees of this type are grown in Australia and Brazil. The bark is smooth throughout, deciduous, bluish grey to apple-pink, sometimes red, and often blotched with all three colors. Younger leaves have a higher percentage of essential oil than mature leaves. *Eucalyptus citriodora* is very similar to Corymbia maculata (also known as Eucalyptus maculata) different only in having slightly narrower crown leaves. Also C. maculata foliage is not lemon scented. Also, it is unlikely that *Eucalyptus citriodora* essential oil is subject to adulteration [115].

Lemon-scented Eucalyptus is one of the only eucalypt species used by the perfume industry. While the oil has limited use directly as a perfume, it is rich in citronellal, which is used to produce other aromatic compounds incorporated extensively in inexpensive perfumes, soaps and disinfectants [116].

Pharmacology and clinical studies for *Eucalyptus citriodora* as bacteriostatic activity towards Staphylococcus aureus. This is due to the synergy between citronellol and citronellal present in the oil [118].

1. **Class:** Aldehydes, alcohol

2. **Family:** *Myrtaceae*

3. **Distillation:** Lemon-scented eucalyptus is steam distilled from the freshly cut leaves and small twigs.

4. **Biochemical:**
   a. alcohol: (+) citronellol (<20%), trans-pinocarveol, geraniol, cis & trans-paramenthane, 3,8-diols
   b. esters: citronellyl, and butyrate
   c. aldehydes: citronellal (>80%)

5. **Uses:**
   a. Antiseptic
   b. Analgesic
   c. Antirheumatic
   d. Antispasmodic
   e. Anti-inflammatory
   f. Antiviral
   g. Bactericidal
   h. Deodorant
   i. Expectorant
   j. Fungicidal
   k. Insecticide/insect repellant
   l. Purifying
   m. Sedative (CNS and cardiac)

6. **Chemical Composition:** The typical chemical composition of lemon-scented eucalyptus essential oil was reported as follows:

    a. α-pinene - 0.14%
    b. citronellal - 80.10%
    c. linalool - 0.66%
    d. isopulegol - 3.41%
    e. iso-isopulegol - 8.51%
    f. β-caryophyllene - 0.39%
    g. citronellol - 4.18%
    h. citronellyl acetate - 0.02%

7. **Systems:**
    a. Integumentary: Provides relief for athlete's foot and other fungal infections, dandruff, herpes, and sores. Also serves as an insecticide.
    b. Respiratory: Provides support for asthma, laryngitis, and sore throat
    c. Muscular/skeletal: Provides support and relief for arthritis (cervical-dorsal, phalanges, and epicondyles), rheumatoid arthritis, rheumatism, muscle and joint aches and pains, especially injuries and sprains.
    d. Cardiovascular: Lowers blood pressure, aids to reduce hypertension, and provides support during recovery from a heart attack.
    e. Immune: Provides support for colds, fevers, and infections. May help with recuperation from long illness. Supports recovery from chicken pox.
    f. Genito-urinary/reproductive: Provides support as a urinary antiseptic and relief for cystitis, vaginitis, and leucorrhea. Increases urine flow.
    g. Central nervous system: Serves to sooth and calm overall system and may ease pain from shingles.

8. **Personality:** *Eucalyptus citriodora* (lemon eucalyptus) personalities have a freshness and exuberance that they bring to everything they do, whether this is in a relationship, at home or at work. If this personality is downhearted, the emotion is occurring because there is too much to do, too many ideas to process, too many places to visit, and

too many people to see even for an extrovert personality. Overall, *citriodora* personalities are fun, creative people. They are enthusiastic, able to handle friends who knock on the door at 2 o'clock in the morning for a cup of coffee, after not seeing them for two years...amazing friends!! [119] The character of *citriodora* is silent, trusting, full of vitality, and harmonious. This oil should be used to support positive attributes: stimulation, concentration, enthusiasm, uplifting, understanding, vitality, creativity, encouragement, positive change, freedom and comforting. This wonderful essential oil will counteract negative attributes such as: sluggishness, emotional crisis, emptiness, confusion, disillusionment, restlessness, fear, despondence, emptiness, and loneliness.[120]

9. **Safety:** Lemon-scented eucalyptus oil is non-toxic, non-irritant and non-sensitizing. However, essential oils in aldehydes such as citral and citronellal may cause sensitization reactions if used undiluted. There are no known contraindications.

10. **Blending:** Top note.

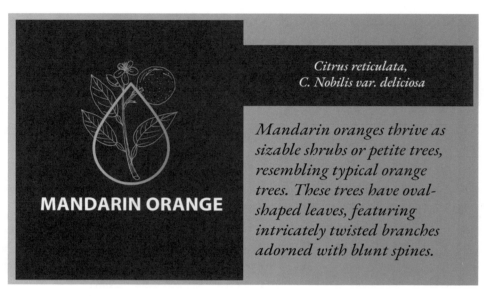

Citrus reticulata,
C. Nobilis var. deliciosa

Mandarin oranges thrive as sizable shrubs or petite trees, resembling typical orange trees. These trees have oval-shaped leaves, featuring intricately twisted branches adorned with blunt spines.

Mandarin Orange
Citrus reticulata, C. Nobilis var. deliciosa

The fruit produced are flat, globe-like shapes that range from 5 to 10 centimeters in diameter. Mandarin orange is normally divided into four groups, each suited to certain climatic and environmental conditions: common, king, willowleaf and satsuma [121].

Mandarin oranges are grown mostly in Europe, and true tangerine, satsuma (easy peel) is cultivated in Sicily. Because this species has many cultivars, mandarin oranges are reportedly the same as tangerines, which are referred to as "satsuma." Varieties produced in the United States tend to be referred to as tangerines. Tangelo is a hybrid between *C. reticulata* and *C. paradisi* [122].

According to Mojay, the mandarin orange is produced by a smaller and more spreading tree than both the sweet and bitter orange trees, with smaller leaves and a more delicately scented peel. [123] In the observations of Shirley and Len Price [123], an aqueous gel containing 5% mandarin produced an immediate hydrating effect on the skin.

Kurt Schnaubelt states that true mandarin is distinguished from tangerine (grown in Florida) by the presence of small of amounts of N-methyl anthranilate, a nitrogen-containing ester, with pronounced relaxing qualities. This compound is not present in tangerine oils. Children universally like this oil, probably

EARTH TREASURES: A FOCUSED JOURNEY INTO THE FOUNDATIONS OF AROMATHERAPY because its aroma is reminiscent of sweets. It is a useful antispasmodic for cardiovascular, digestive, and respiratory systems. It soothes restlessness, especially in hyperactive children and calms the activity of sympathetic nervous system. It ameliorates stubborn patterns of insomnia and is particularly effective in combination with sweet orange essential oil. His preferred mode of use is topical through massage and inhalation. According to Schnaubelt, the highest quality and most effective oil is organic, although organic is not readily or consistently available in the world market [125].

Apart from its use in aromatherapy, mandarin oil is extensively used in flavors, where it gives interesting modifications with sweet and bitter orange oils, grapefruit, and lime oil in flavor compositions for soft drinks, candy, and liqueurs. In France, mandarin oil is considered the children's remedy and is used to relieve tummy upsets of babies and children. Mandarin oil is recommended for soothing restlessness, especially in hyperactive children. [126]

1. **Class**: Aldehyde

2. **Family**: *Rutaceae*

3. **Distillation**: Expressed from the fruit rind of *C. reticulata.*

4. **Biochemical**:
    a. Monoterpenes: d-limonene (up to 75%), seen with up to 90% may indicate addition of sweet orange essential oil). y-terpinene, α-pinene, myrcene.
    b. Alcohols: nonanol, octanol, geraniol
    c. Monoterpenols: citronellol, linalool
    d. Esters: benzul acetate
    e. Nitrogen compounds: methyl-n-methyl anthranilate (>1%)
    f. Aldehydes: decanal, citral, citronellal, coumarins and furocoumarins.

5. **Uses**:
    a. Antifungal
    b. Antiseptic

c. Antispasmodic
d. Bactericide
e. Carminative
f. Cholagogue
g. Depurative
h. Digestive
i. Diuretic
j. Sedative (tranquilizer)
k. Stimulant (lymphatic)
l. Tonic (digestive carminative)

6. **Chemical composition**: A typical chemical composition of mandarin is reported as follows: [121]
   a. α-thujone – 0.76 - 0.96%
   b. α-pinene – 2.12 - 2.54%
   c. sabinene – 0.24 - 0.29%
   d. β-pinene – 0.25 - 1.82%
   e. myrcene – 1.69 - 1.77%
   f. limonene – 67.92 - 74.00%
   g. y-terpinolene – 16.78 - 21.02%
   h. linalool – 0.05 - 0.16%
   i. citronellal – 0.02 - 0.04%
   j. terpinen-4-ol – 0.02 - 0.06%
   k. nerol – 0.01 - 0.02%
   l. geranial – 0.03 - 0.06%

7. **Systems**:
   a. Integumentary: Serves as a skin toner, controls acne, and supports congested oil and combination skin. Works great as a moisturizer, softens dry skin, and reduces the appearance of scars and stretch marks. Provides support for cellulite.
   b. Respiratory: Relieves difficulty in breathing.
   c. Muscular/skeletal: Relieves muscle spasms.
   d. Cardiovascular/lymphatic: Provides support for cardiovascular erethism. Increases lymphatic circulation and may aid in detoxification.

e. Immune: Serves as an immunostimulant.

f. Digestive: Provides relief from indigestion, gastritis, dyspepsia, aerophagy, hiccups, constipation, and intestinal challenges.

g. Genito-urinary/reproductive: Increases urine flow and support for edema due to simple water retention. Provides support for PMS, and menstrual cramps.

h. Central nervous system: aids sensitivities, calms excitations, insomnia (especially nervous origin), tension, nervousness, and restlessness. Brings child-like energy and provides support for establishing routines.

8. **Personality**: The mandarin personality is sweet, gentle, kind and loving—one of the softest personalities. Their kindness is extended to all living, breathing things including plants, fish, animals, humans as well as to inanimate objects like the teddy bear that was precious to them as a child. Mandarin characters are very uplifting and can "gladden the old man's heart" and are often taking care of the older generation. Unfortunate, this soft personality can become hysterical at the slightest thing and is often compulsive about cleanliness, both personal and domestic. This personality is prone to nightmares and may experience paralyzing fear out of all proportion – afraid to meet people, afraid of life, and struggling with unnecessary grief. The character for mandarin is gentle, peaceful, revitalizing, and sympathetic. This oil can be used to encourage these positive attributes: calm, uplifted spirit, refreshment, inspiration, soothing, brightness, integrity, and tranquility. This essential oil counteracts these negative attributes: anxiety, depression, grief, abusive behavior, emptiness, focus on the past, overexcitability, isolation, and emotional trauma. [127]

9. **Safety**: Tested at low dose, nontoxic, non-irritating, non-sensitizing. Older oxidized oils or those with high d-limonene increases potential for sensitization. Phototoxic.

10. **Blending**: Top/middle note.

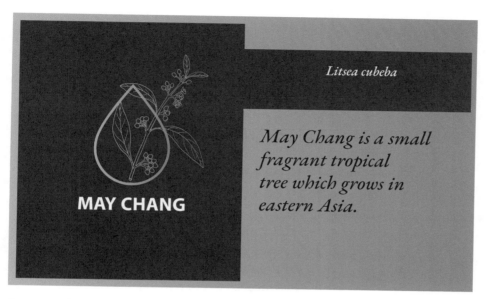

Litsea cubeba

May Chang is a small fragrant tropical tree which grows in eastern Asia.

May Chang
Litsea cubeba

China is the largest producer of May Chang oil. Most oil suppliers refer to May Chang by its botanical name *Litsea cubeba*. It has been known for its fragrant flowers, fruit, and leave for a long time. The small fruit resembles the cubeb pepper, thus the scientific name. It was not until the 1950s that may chang essential oil was recognized. While it is often compared with lemongrass, its odor is considered to be finer, more lemon-like and less fatty [128].

On the pharmacological applications, Robert Tisserand and Tony Balacs cite clinical trials using may chang for the treatment of experimentally induced cardiac arrhythmias. It was compared with propranolol (a beta-blocker, antihypertensive, and anti-angina drug). The test results confirmed Litsea cubeba to reduce arrhythmias from 15 minutes to 6.5 minutes compared to propranolol, which reduced the arrhythmia time from 15 minutes to 0.6 minutes.[129]

1. **Class**: Aldehyde

2. **Family**: *Lauraceae*

3. **Distillation**: May Chang essential oil is steam distilled from the small, pepper-like fruits

4. **Biochemical:**
    a. Monoterpenes: (<14%): myrcene, limonene
    b. Sesquiterpenes: (<1%): β-caryophyllene
    c. Alcohols: linalool, α-terpineol, citronellol, neral, geraniol
    d. Esters: Linalyl acetate, terpenyl, neryl, geranyl
    e. Aldehydes (approx. 85%): citrals: neral (>35%), geranial (<39%), citronellal
    f. Ketones: methyl heptenone

5. **Uses**:
    a. Antidepressant
    b. Anti-inflammatory
    c. Antiseptic
    d. Astringent
    e. Anti-infectious
    f. Bactericide
    g. Carminative
    h. Deodorant
    i. Disinfectant
    j. Galactagogue
    k. Insecticidal
    l. Stimulant
    m. Sedative Tonic (digestive)

6. **Chemical composition**: A typical chemical composition of May Chang is reported as follows: [128]
    a. α-pinene - 0.87%
    b. β-pinene – 0.39%
    c. myrcene - 3.04%
    d. limonene – 8.38%
    e. neral – 33.80%
    f. geranial – 40.61%
    g. nerol – 1.09%
    h. geraniol – 1.58%
    i. linalool – 1.7%
    j. linalyl acetate – 1.65%
    k. caryophyllene – 0.51%

May Chang is chemically similar to lemongrass, melissa and other essential oils rich in citral. Citral comprises approximately 75% of May chang essential oil and contains two isomers: neral and geranial [130].

7. **Systems**:
    a. Integumentary: Provides support for blemishes, excessively oily skin, and hair health. Can also provide relief for acne, dermatitis, fungal infections. Serves as an insect repellant (use only as in a dilution because it is a possible irritant).
    b. Respiratory: Serves as an effective tonic, applied through asthma bronco-dilator. Effective in a diffuser for room cleaning in combination with pines and eucalyptus.
    c. Cardiovascular: Serves as a heart tonic. May support high blood pressure, coronary heart disease, and arteriosclerosis. May also support reduction of tumors.
    d. Digestive: Provides relief from flatulence, nausea, anorexia, gastro-duodenal ulcers, and indigestion.
    e. Genito-urinary/reproductive: Increases milk secretion.
    f. Central nervous system: Supports by uplifting and stimulating spirits and energy. Combats fatigue, lethargy, insomnia, anxiety, and nervous depression.

8. **Personality**: May Chang is categorized as a "fruitie" personality, with aspirations to feel harmony, have security, respect, and approval within themselves. "Fruities" are self-aware, emotionally balanced, and are usually very kind, happy people. They are generally well-liked because they radiate positivity and friendliness. May chang personalities fall into this category, and in general, their personalities are compliant, dutiful, conventional, organized, respectful, jovial, and willing to please. You cannot define a "fruitie" as in introvert or extrovert because they swing between the two in equal

proportions. May Chang personalities need to express themselves and are very creative in relationships. They have a very independent nature, great faith in themselves, and tremendous courage. When the May Chang "fruitie" person is imbalanced, they become tired, and faded, defensive, and indecisive. Self-criticism takes over, along with self-sacrifice and servility and in some cases, masochistic actions. Disheartened with life and people, they stagnate and stay at home becoming increasingly impatient, touchy, and oversensitive, and aggressive if people try to help [131].

According to Battaglia, may chang essential oil helps to promote optimisms, vision, and foresight whenever there is pessimism, negative thinking, and loss of vision. [132] According to Robbi Zeck, Litsea cubeba essential oil ranges from successful to despairing when imbalanced. They shine their incandescent light on all things like shadows dancing on water. When is despair and at your wits end ask yourself " *Who would I be without these thoughts of despair*?" Question yourself relentlessly. Be interested in yourself!" [133]

9. **Safety**: Tisserand recommends a dermal maximum of 0.8% to void skin sensitization. This is based on the International Fragrance Association (IFRA) maximum for citral of 0.6% for body oils and lotions and 75% citral content. He recommends a daily oral maximum in pregnancy of 56 mg. This is based on 74% citral content, with dermal and oral citral limited of 0.6% and 0.6mg/kg [134].

    According to Sheppard-Hanger, it was tested at low dose indicating non-toxic, possible skin irritant, and possible sensitization. This essential oil has a very strong scent. [135]

10. **Blending**: Top note.

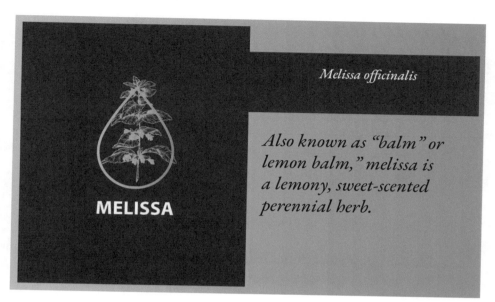

Melissa officinalis

Also known as "balm" or lemon balm," melissa is a lemony, sweet-scented perennial herb.

Melissa
Melissa officinalis

Growing between 30 and 60 centimeters (11 to 23 inches tall) with bright-green, oval-to-heart- shaped leaves and small, loose clusters of white, pink or yellowish flowers. Native to the Mediterranean, melissa is now cultivated in gardens in the world over. Revered since ancient times, its name derives from the Greek melittena, or "honeybee" because according to Dioscorides, "The bees do delight in the herb." Cultivated as a plant to attract bees, its abundant nectar helps to produce some of the very best honey. A great deal of melissa oil currently being sold is not essential oil derived from the true *Melissa officinalis*. Rather, it is often a blend of lemongrass and citronella, together with naturally derived chemicals similar to the chemical constituent of the real product. [136]

According to Dr. Kurt Schnaubelt, true melissa essential oil is the most expensive essential oil on the market. Production is costly, as the yield is low and distillation often difficult. It is highly effective on herpes lesions, but other less expensive oils can also be effective. Melissa essential oil is a powerful sedative, relaxing the body for easier sleep and ameliorating anger in crisis or trauma. This oil should be highly diluted to utilize its anti-inflammatory properties. He warns against skin tolerance, as it may vary. Dr. Schnaubelt's preferred mode of use is internal, topical, or as a fragrance, but itself and in compositions. The quality is available in genuine and authentic quality, but clever substitutes abound also. [137]

Melissa oil is distilled in the South of France, Germany, Italy, and Spain. However, the total production of genuine melissa oil is only a fraction of the quantity commercially offered. Melissa oil has the dubious reputation of being one of the most frequently adulterated essential oils. [138]

A spiritual balm created with melissa essential oil by combining lemon peel, nutmeg, angelica root, and other herbs and spices became popular under the name of "carmelite water." This blend was considered beneficial for the treatment of nervous headaches, digestive problems, and neuralgic affections. [139]

1. **Class**: Aldehydes, sesquiterpenes

2. **Family**: *Lamiaceae* or *Labiatae*

3. **Distillation**: Melissa oil is steam distilled from the leaves and flowering tops of *M. officinalis*.

4. **Biochemical**:
   a. Monoterpenes: iso & trans-ocimenes
   b. Sesquiterpenes: α-cubebene, α-copaene, β-bourbonene, β-caryophyllene (>7%), α-humulene, germacrene D (>5%)
   c. Alcohols: 1-octene-3-ol, cis-3-hexanol, Linalool, nerol, geraniol, citronellol, α-terpineol, terpinen-4-ol, 10-pei-α-cadinol, caryophyllenol, farnesol
   d. Esters: geranyl, neryl, linalyl & citronellyl acetates
   e. Oxides: 1,8 cineol, caryophyllene oxide
   f. Aldehydes: citrals: neral (>16%), geranial (>15%) citronellal and α-cyclocitral
   g. Coumarin: aesculetin - Also eugenol.

5. **Uses**:
   a. Antiallergenic
   b. Antidepressant
   c. Antihistaminic
   d. Anti-inflammatory
   e. Antispasmodic
   f. Antiviral
   g. Antibacterial

    h.   Antifungal
    i.   Bactericidal
    j.   Carminative
    k.   Choleretic
    l.   Cordial
    m.   Diaphoretic
    n.   Digestive
    o.   Emmenagogues
    p.   Febrifuge
    q.   Hypotensive
    r.   Hypnotic (sedative, nervous)
    s.   Insect repellant
    t.   Nervine
    u.   Stimulant (muscular)
    v.   Sedative
    w.   Sudorific
    x.   Tonic (uterine, cardiac)
    y.   Vermifuge

6. **Chemical composition**: A typical chemical composition of melissa oil is reported as follows: [140]
    a.   trans-ocimene – 0.2%
    b.   cis-ocimene – 0.1%
    c.   methyl heptenone – 0.6%
    d.   3-octanone – 0.6%
    e.   cis-3-hexanol – 0.1%
    f.   3-octanol – 0.1%
    g.   1-octen-3-ol – 1.3%
    h.   copaene – 4.0%
    i.   citronellal – 0.7%
    j.   linalool – 0.4%
    k.   β-bourbonene – 0.3%
    l.   caryophyllene – 9.5%
    m.   α-humulene – 0.2%
    n.   neral – 24.1%
    o.   germacrene d – 4.2%
    p.   geranial – 37.2%
    q.   geranyl acetate – 0.5%

r.   d-cadinene – 1.1%
s.   y-cadinene – 1.0%
t.   nerol – 0.1%
u.   geraniol – 0.1%

7. **Systems:**
   a. Integumentary: Provides support for oily skin, acne, allergies, insect bites, cold sores, herpes, fungal infections, and wounds. May also reduce blood flow; however, there is no specific research testing for wounds and blood flow coagulation.
   b. Respiratory: Provides support for asthma, bronchitis, chronic coughs, colds (with headache), and rapid breathing.
   c. Muscular/skeletal: Serves as a tonic for muscle spasm, fatigue, and rheumatism pain in low doses.
   d. Cardiovascular/lymphatic system: Calms circulation, strengthens and slows heart, lowers blood pressures, and eases palpitations due to crisis. Provides calming effect for unusual stimulation, excitation, fear.
   e. Immune: Excellent support for colds, flu, fevers, strep infections, and viral infections including herpes simplex.
   f. Digestive: Provides support for colic, nausea, vomiting, stomach cramps, and indigestion. Stimulates liver and provides liver and gallbladder support.
   g. Genito-urinary/reproductive: Provides support for menstrual pain and problems with fertility. Balances hormones and regulates menstrual cycle.
   h. Central nervous system: Relieves anxiety, depression, hypertension, insomnia and migraines. Provides support for hysterics, nervous crisis, tension, and vertigo. Is calming, and uplifting. Dispels fear, shock and grief. May help with anger and brings acceptance and understanding. May help to deal with past lives.

8. **Personality**: Melissa personality is bubbly, fizzy, full of energy, and usually delightful with a multitude of interests and activities. This personality is not only highly organized, but they also have such a love of life that even one second is too precious too waste. Melissa personalities attract jealousy, spitefulness, and unadventurous souls who feed off their vivacious, outgoing nature and admire their control of life. The trouble is these people want to tame the melissa personality to make her (or him) more like themselves. Throughout all of this, the melissa personality always tries to find the good side in people. The character of melissa would be hypnotic, empowering, mesmerizing, sagacious. Melissa oil encourages these positive attributes: inspiration, creativity, stillness, inner vision, aspirations, idealism, sensuality, vision, discovery and truthfulness. Melissa oil counteracts these negative attributes: hysteria, nervousness, irritability, addictions, withdrawal, loneliness, illusions, disillusionment, longings, obsessions, trauma, emotional wounds, misery, and anguish [140].

   Robbi Zeck likes to describe the melissa oil personality as a beam of light on a dark winter's day, softening extreme emotion, easing resentment, gladdening the heart and engaging the soul in its own rhythm. Reaching inward, caressing the inner being, the warm radiance of melissa oil directs the spirit toward mindful reflection on all that you have to be grateful for. Breath in the fresh, light scent of melissa oil and let gratitude open you to the treasures of your heart. [142]

9. **Safety**: Melissa oil is non-toxic. However, according to Battaglia, care must be taken as the oil is a possible sensitizer and dermal irritant. Caution must also be taken when choosing suppliers as this is a frequently adulterated essential oil.

10. **Blending**: Middle note.

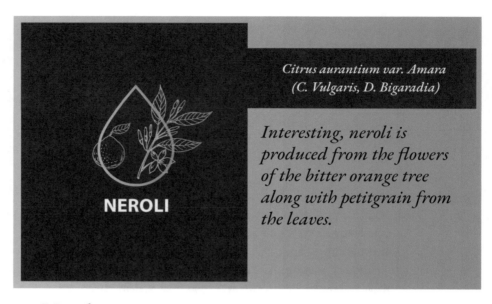

Citrus aurantium var. Amara
(C. Vulgaris, D. Bigaradia)

Interesting, neroli is produced from the flowers of the bitter orange tree along with petitgrain from the leaves.

Neroli
Citrus aurantium var. Amara (C. vulgaris, C. bigaradia)

It is commonly known as orange flower, orange blossom, and neroli bigarade. The bitter orange is an evergreen tree with long but not sharp spines and very fragrant flowers. It is native to southern China and India. Neroli bigarade is produced in the south of France, Italy, Tunisia, Morocco, Haiti, Guinea, and Algeria. The essential oil can often be difficult to obtain and expensive; thus, synthetic substances are often commercially sold. These synthetic chemicals should be avoided in aromatherapy, as they will not provide the same healing essence as the natural oil. The bitter orange was first cultivated in the Mediterranean by Arabs in the 10th and 11th centuries. The oil was first distilled in the early 16th century, and it was named after the 17th century Italian princess of Nerola. Anna Maria De LaTremoille, who wore the oil in her gloves. [143]

According to Fischer-Rizzi, neroli has always been one the of the most expensive oils. One ton of orange blossoms is needed to produce a single quart of oil, and the blossoms must be picked by hand. The essential oil neroli bigarade is superior when compared to oil from sweet orange blossom oil (C. *sinensis*). It is helpful for treating depression and used very similarly as a "rescue remedy" in Bach Flower therapy. [144]

Neroli was employed as a scent by the prostitutes of Madrid, so they would be recognized by its aroma. On the other hand, the blossoms were worn as a wedding headdress and carried as a bouquet, symbolizing purity and virginity. [145] This usage would indicate that the prostitutes were highly paid and respected for their work during this time, suggesting that they were healthy and perhaps provided services to the upper class.

Dr. Kurt Schnaubelt suggests that neroli essential oil is soothing and strengthening element in perfume compositions for exhausted nervous types. It facilitates birthing and eases post-partum depression. It is a hepatic and pancreatic stimulant containing the dimeric form (meaning chemistry of a molecule composed of two identical simpler molecules – monomers – and ocimene are a group of isometric hydrocarbons) of ocimene, a youth hormone. This composition may explain its effectiveness in preventing stretch marks. His preferred mode of use is topical and as a perfume. He states that sadly, importers are often unwilling to pay the real price for this oil and revert to clever marketing of cheaper substitutes. [146]

1. **Class**: Monoterpenes

2. **Family**: *Rutaceae*

3. **Distillation**: Neroli essential oil is obtained from the freshly picked flowers of *C. aurantium*, subspecies *amara* by steam distillation

4. **Biochemical**:
    a. Monoterpenes: (90 – 92%): d-limonene, terpinolene, myrcene, camphene, pinene, ocimene, cymene
    b. Alcohols: linalool (+)-α-terpineol, citronellol, nerol, geraniol
    c. Esters:(2%): geranyl acetate, neryl acetate, citronellyl and linalyl acetate, methyl anthranilate
    d. Aldehydes (0.8 - 7%): nonanal, decanal, undecenal, dodecanal, geranial, neral, citronellal
    e. Coumarins & furocoumarins (0.90%): auraptene, auraptenol, bergaptene, bergaptol, scoparone, citroptene

5. **Uses:**
   a. Anticoagulant
   b. Antidepressant
   c. Anti-inflammatory
   d. Antiseptic
   e. Antispasmodic
   f. Bactericidal
   g. Carminative
   h. Cicatrizant
   i. Cordial
   j. Deodorant
   k. Digestive
   l. Febrifuge
   m. Fungicidal
   n. Hypotensive
   o. Nervine
   p. Sedative (mild)
   q. Tonic (nervous system)

6. **Chemical composition**: A typical chemical composition of neroli is reported as follows:[147]
   a. α-pinene – 4.6%
   b. camphene – 5.5%
   c. sabinene – 2.5%
   d. β-pinene – 8.67%
   e. myrcene – 2.1%
   f. 8-3-carene – 2.46%
   g. limonene – 22.43%
   h. terpinene – 4.14%
   i. a-terpineol – 1.87%
   j. linalool – 2.52%
   k. linalyl acetate – 0.87%
   l. geraniol – 1.02%
   m. nerol – 6.97%
   n. citronellol – 1.87%
   o. citral – 2.41%
   p. β-citral – 1.87%
   q. methyl anthranilate – 1.89%

7. **Systems**:
    a. Integumentary: Excellent support for dry dull, oily, and congested skin including wrinkles and acne. Works well with mouth ulcers. Strengthens and softens epidermis. Stimulates nerve endings and melanocyte, including pigment development and circulation. Aids hydration. Calms gland functions. Increases hydrolipid layer, which may help skin from drying out. Supports regeneration of cells and serves as a preventative for stretch marks.
    b. Respiratory: Supports bronchitis and chills.
    c. Muscular/skeletal: Provides support for sore muscles and bones. Used in combined with collagen to repair the bones and tissue.
    d. Cardiovascular/lymphatic: Increases circulation, raises blood pressure, promotes warmth, and eases palpitations. Serves as an anticoagulant and blood thinner.
    e. Immune: Serves as an immunostimulant. Excellent support for colds flu, chills, and fever
    f. Digestive: Supports kidney and gallbladder action. Aids with constipation, dyspepsia, spasm, edema (simple water retention), and high cholesterol. Raises blood sugar; increases intestinal resorption; and relaxes and soothes muscle cells in intestines and digestive glands.
    g. Endocrine: Stimulates all anterior love hormones and gonadotropic hormones, including sex hormones, growth hormones, and pigmentation. Activates the connecting organs and stimulates the adrenal medulla (adrenaline, noradrenaline).
    h. Genito-urinary/reproductive: Relaxes uterus, smooths muscles, and aids post-partum depression.
    i. Central nervous system: Activates sympathetic nervous system and adrenal medulla. Eases anxiety and insomnia (due to anxiety). Soothes

nervous stomach and dispels tension and stress. Aids in need for warmth, revives interest in life, and energizes mental clarity and concentration on all levels.

8. **Personality**: Neroli, also known as orange blossom, is one of the most spiritual personalities – another angel, like chamomile roman. Neroli types are happiest when searching the mysteries of life as a hobby. Saddened by the lack of understanding in the world today, then can turn to being supersensitive souls. Neroli personalities can be very deep emotionally and if in a negative frame of mind, are easily angered, usually with the "you just don't understand" kind of line. [148]. The character of neroli is spiritual, pure, loving, and peaceful. Neroli oils encourages these positive attributes: lightness, lifting of sorrows, spirituality, connection, completeness, joy, understanding, calm, stable, peaceful. Neroli oil counteracts these negative attributes: anxiety, stress, tension, shock, emotional crisis, sadness, longing, panic, grief, childhood abuse, adult abuse, depression, hopelessness, and fear.

   Zeck says that neroli encourages trusting the emotional intelligence that guides choices and is an essential component of natural expression. The delightfully sweet scent of neroli fosters these choices, building bridges between the inner realms where renewed life force takes place. [149]

9. **Safety**: Tested as non-toxic, non-irritating. However, older, oxidized oils or those with high d-limonene increase the potential for sensitization. Prolonged use and/or high dose may irritate sensitive skin.

10. **Blending**: Top note.

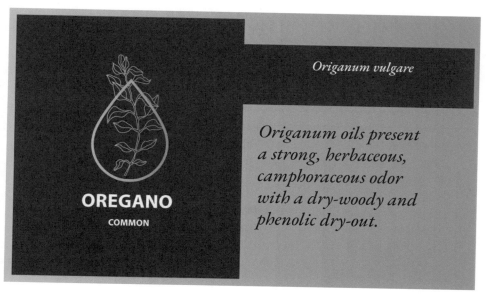

Origanum vulgare

Origanum oils present a strong, herbaceous, camphoraceous odor with a dry-woody and phenolic dry-out.

Oregano, Common
Origanum vulgare

Oregano is a flowering herb plant with has several plant species native to Europe. The most commonly used plants are:
1)   *Thymus capitatus*
2)   *Origanum vulgare*
3)   *Origanum smyrnaceum*
4)   *Origanum maru*

According to Sylla-Sheppard-Hanger, the *O. vulgare var. viride* contains up to 50% thymol, which is a skin irritant. *O. dictamnus* is grown and harvested from areas in Dittany, Greece, and Crete near the Middle East. Grown in the same area, *O. syriacum* was considered hyssop, referenced in the Bible at Jesus' crucifixion. [150]

Origanum vulgare is the true oregano of the garden herb, which has been historically used as a medicine and culinary herb. The main constituents in oregano oil are carvacrol and thymol. Both constituents are phenols that contribute to oregano's properties as a skin irritant and mucous membrane irritant [151].

According to Len and Shirley Price, when the hydroxyl group attaches itself to a carbon in an aromatic (also known as phenyl and/or benzene) ring, the resulting molecule is known as a phenol, which is an aromatic alcohol with powerful effects. Phenols also have names which end in "-ol" (e.g., carvacrol).

To discriminate between the two classes, it is necessary to learn the names of the most important members in each group. Phenols, like alcohols, are antiseptic and bactericidal. Because they stimulate both the nervous system (making them effective against depressive illness) and the immune system, they activate the body's own healing process. However, because the -OH molecule is attached to a ring rather than to a chain molecule, aromatic phenols, unlike the aliphatic alcohols, can be toxic to the liver and irritant to the skin if used in substantial amounts or for a long period. Oregano owes its value in the pharmaceutical field almost entirely to the antiseptic and germicidal properties of its phenolic content. [152]

Observations with *Origanum vulgare subsp. viride* (Greek oregano/green oregano) was that it was effective against three strains of *Candida albicans*. The main component of carvacrol and emulsified oregano oil was used successfully via oral administration (with capsules) to treat patients having enteric parasites. [153]

Kurt Schnaubelt states that in 1910, William Martindale [154] demonstrated that oregano essential oil is the strongest plant-derived antiseptic known to date. Oregano is twenty-five to seventy-six times more active than isolated phenol on the coli bacillus. The coli bacillus is Gram negative (often written Gram -) bacillus or rod-shaped bacillus. *Escherichia coli* (*e. coli*) has a double-stranded, circular DNA genome containing 4.6 million base pairs that have been completely sequenced. Using a broad-based assessment of antibacterial and antifungal properties with the aromatogram technique, the results show that oregano has one of the broadest overall spectrums of action. And in 1987, Deininger and Lembke demonstrated the antiviral activity of this essential oil and its isolated components. [155] The ability of plants to influence the hormonal balance of other organisms is not limited to toxins and poisons but includes the creation of an allure or symbiotic advantage of other species such as belladonna and digitoxin from foxglove. This aspect is obvious in the specific interactions between sesquiterpenes and human receptor sites, which are currently being researched. Oregano falls into this category with components that include mono- and sesquiterpenes. [156]

Similar to thyme, Oregano essential oil has a large spectrum of antibacterial, antifungal and antiparasitic action and energizes during general asthenia. Oregano may not have the self-asserting influence on the thymus gland, which is alluded to in the name of thyme. Dr. Schnaubelt's preferred mode of use is internally, ideally diluted in vegetable oil and in capsules. The quality is often industrial and variable, but genuine products are available. [156]

1. **Class**: Phenol

2. **Family**: *Labiatae*

3. **Distillation**: Steam distilled from the dried, flowering plants.

4. **Biochemical**:
    a. Monoterpenes & sesquiterpenes: cymene, pinene, caryophyllene, bisabolene, terpinene
    b. Alcohol: linalool, borneol
    c. Esters: geranyl acetate, linalyl acetate
    d. Phenols: carvacrol, thymol-P

5. **Uses**:
    a. Analgesic (pain relief)
    b. Anti-inflammatory
    c. Antibacterial
    d. Antidepressant
    e. Antifungal
    f. Antioxidant
    g. Antimicrobial
    h. Antiseptic
    i. Antiviral
    j. Anti-infectious
    k. Antispasmodic
    l. Antiallergenic,
    m. Antirheumatic
    n. Antitoxic
    o. Bactericidal
    p. Bechic
    q. Carminative
    r. Choleretic
    s. Cytophylactic
    t. Diaphoretic
    u. Diuretic
    v. Disinfectant
    w. Dyspepsia

x. Emmenagogue
y. Eczema
z. Expectorant
aa. Febrifuge
ab. Fungicidal
ac. Hepatic
ad. Indigestion
ae. Laxative
af. Immune stimulant
ag. Parasiticide
ah. Nerve tonic
ai. Removes warts
aj. Rubefacient
ak. Splenic
al. Stimulant
am. Stomachic
an. Sudorific
ao. Tonic
ap. Vulnerary

6. **Chemical composition**: A typical chemical composition of oregano is reported as follows:
   a. carvacrol – 14.0%
   b. thymol – 12%
   c. p-cymene – 3.0%
   d. cis-ocimene – 13.5%
   e. caryophyllene – 9.2%
   f. linalool – 3.0%

7. **Systems**:
   a. Integumentary: Provides support for infected cuts and wounds. Also combats parasites.
   b. Respiratory: Works well with asthma, colds, bronchitis, catarrh, and whopping cough
   c. Muscular/skeletal: Provides relief from rheumatism and muscle pain.
   d. Immune: Provides support for colds, flu, and infections.

e.   Digestive: Sooths nervous stomach disorders, stimulates liver and spleen, calms intestinal spasms and flatulence, and stimulates appetite. May support with aerophagia (gulping of air).

f.   Genito-urinary/reproductive: Provides support for period pains. Serves as an excellent diuretic. Caution interacts with hormones (when creating a blend for a PMS or menopausal/andro-pausal person.

g.   Central nervous system: Excellent stimulant and nerve tonic. Revives the senses. Possibility of easing deafness, pain, noise in ears. Helpful with migraines, and facial tics. Relieves imaginary diseases and mental psychopathic conditions, producing a feeling of well-being.

8.   **Personality**: Oregano essential oil reduces insecurity and encourages a general feeling of well-being. It promotes a sense of security. [157]. Battaglia states as a "herbie" personality, it gives confidence, energy and focus to those who use it. Kurt Schnaubelt states that oregano can be an irritant to specific individuals based on their unique disposition. [158]. With oregano and thyme being similar in constituents, Mojay states that is it a Yang (male) oil and is further reflected in its invigorating mental-emotional affects. It is fortifying and uplifting as it is indicated for nervous debility and chronic anxiety. It can be compared to Thor, the god of thunderstorms, a generous Germanic deity – a gentle giant – who broke into a thunderous range when provoked. With his magic hammer in hand, he makes a fitting symbol of the assertiveness and bravery that this oil imparts. [159]

9.   **Safety**: Avoid use during pregnancy and lactation [160]. Also avoid using for babies and children. Oregano may negatively affect embryonic development and encourage fetal cell death according to animal research. It may also interact with aspirin, blood pressure, antiplatelet, and

anticoagulant medications, which increases the risk of bleeding and is of particular concern for anyone with bleeding disorders. Oregano essential oil may interact with antibiotics and possibly enhance their effects. It may also interact with diabetic medications and cause low blood-sugar levels. It may irritate mucous membranes including eyes, mouth, nasal passages, vagina, and rectum. [161] Oregano oil is not recommended for use on person with hypersensitive skin, diseased or damaged skin, or children under 2 years of age. [162] This aromatic medicine is hepatotoxic in large doses.

10. **Blending**: Mild, medium note.

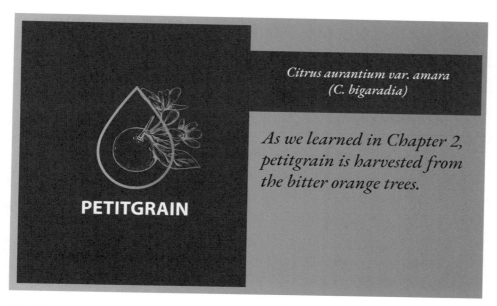

Citrus aurantium var. amara (C. bigaradia)

As we learned in Chapter 2, petitgrain is harvested from the bitter orange trees.

Petitgrain
Citrus aurantium var. amara (C. bigaradia)

Many essential oils are produced from the entire plant; however, some oils are produced from specific parts of the plant (leaves, flowers, bark or stem) because the essential oil varies in quality and chemistry according to the part used for production. Bitter orange, also known at petitgrain sur fleur, is a classic example of a tree from which three types of essential oils are produced.

Petitgrain oil is a pale yellow or amber-colored liquid of pleasant, fresh-floral, and sweet odor that is reminiscent of orange flowers with a slightly woody-herbaceous undertone and a very faint but sweet floral dry-out. [163] It is an evergreen tree with long but not very sharp spines and very fragrant flowers. It is a native of southern China and north-eastern India. The tree is cultivated in mild, temperate, semitropical, and tropical areas of the world such as the south of France, Italy, Algeria, Tunisia, Morocco, Spain, west Africa, and Paraguay. The oil produced from Paraguay is referred to as petitgrain Paraguay and the oil from France is referred to as petitgrain bigarade.

It has been suggested that the oil from France is of superior quality because the French producers are careful to use only the leaf and not include any of the wooden branches, nor any small unripe fruit. [164]

1. **Class**: Ester, alcohol, monoterpene

2. **Family**: *Rutaceae*

3. **Distillation**: Steam distilled from the dried, flowering plants.

4. **Biochemical**:
    a. Essential oil:
        i. Monoterpenes: (10%): β-myrcene, cis & trans-ocimene, paracymene, paracymene, d-limonene, camphene, α-terpinene, β-pinene
        ii. Sesquiterpenes: β-caryophyllene, farnesene
        iii. Alcohols: (40%): (+) & (-)-linalool (20%), (+)-a-terpineol, nerol, geraniol Esters: (5.0-80%): linalyl acetate (up to 55%), neryl acetate, terpenyl, and geranyl acetate
        iv. Nitrogen compounds: methyl anthranilate
        v. Aldehyde: citral

    b. Hydrolat:
        i. Methyl anthranilate

5. **Uses**:
    a. Antiseptic
    b. Antispasmodic
    c. Anti-infectious
    d. Anti-inflammative
    e. Antibacterial (staph, pneumococcus)
    f. Deodorant
    g. Nervine (balances nervous system/sedation and stimulation)
    h. Stomachic (digestive stimulant)
    i. Sedative

6. **Chemical composition**: A typical chemical composition of petitgrain is reported as follows: [165]
   a. geranial - 2.33%
   b. linalool - 27.95%
   c. nerol – 1.015
   d. α-terpineol – 7.55%
   e. geranyl acetate - 2.61%
   f. linalyl acetate – 44.29%
   g. myrcene – 5.36%
   h. neryl acetate – 0.55%
   i. trans-ocimene – 3.32%

The most important constituent of petitgrain which defines quality is linalyl acetate. Petitgrain Paraguay oil has a lower ester and higher alcohol content than the petitgrain bigarade of French origin. [165]

7. **Systems**:
   a. Integumentary: Provides support for dry acne, boils, oily skin, and hair. Also supports dry skin and tones. Serves as an excellent deodorant to address excessive perspiration
   b. Respiratory: Eases breathing and supports all respiratory infections, especially via back massage. Eases nervous asthma. Petitgrain is also a cicatrizant, which is a Portuguese word meaning healing, suggesting tissue and regeneration possibilities.
   c. Muscular/skeletal: Relaxes muscle spasm (of the nervous origin) and increases muscle tone. May support joint inflammation, including inflammation resulting from arthritis and rheumatism
   d. Cardiovascular/lymphatic: Eases palpitations and cardiovascular spasms. Improves arterial circulation.
   e. Immune: Servers as an immune stimulant.
   f. Digestive: Provides support for dyspepsia, gas,

and painful digestion. Calms stomach muscles and tones digestive system. May be useful in chronic hepatitis.

g.   Central nervous system: Provides support for insomnia. Balances central nervous system from exhaustion. Serves as one of the best remedies for these challenges. Provides support for stress, mental fatigue, panic, and anger. Refreshes the mind, gives mental clarity, eases disharmony, and revives the body.

8.   **Personality**: The petitgrain personality appears to be in control, capable and never fazed, but is often underestimated. Their qualities are not always given the deserved recognition. Petitgrain personalities are not dull individuals and can make stimulating company if given the chance. They tend to be good conversationalists who are interested in other people's opinions... or at least they give that impression, being too polite to do otherwise. When they are feeling negative, they become disillusioned with the general lack of concern for human life expressed in this world and often try to alleviate these feelings by doing something positive themselves, no matter how small. [166] The character of petitgrain would be revitalizing, balancing, restoring, clarifying. This oil encourages these positive attributes: harmony, uplifted spirit, inner vision, strength, self-confidence, optimism. This essential oil counteracts these negative attributes: disharmony, confusion, difficulty, mental fatigue, nervous exhaustion, insomnia, disappointment, betrayal, anger, irrationality, introversion, and pessimism.[166].

According to Robbi Zeck, the fresh stimulating aroma of petitgrain drifts across the pathways of the conscious mind, encouraging memories to lead to deeper awakening. Memories create the blueprint of individual expression. Petitgrain oil opens the memory, gaining entrance to the place within consciousness where far-off memories reside. Through surrender to the awareness that is beyond conscious thought, this frontier can bring new insights to illuminate each path through life. [168]

9. **Safety**: Tested at low dosages, non-toxic, non-irritant, non-sensitizing, non-phototoxic. A cross sensitivity is reported with existing allergic reactions to balsams.

10. **Blending**: Middle to top note.

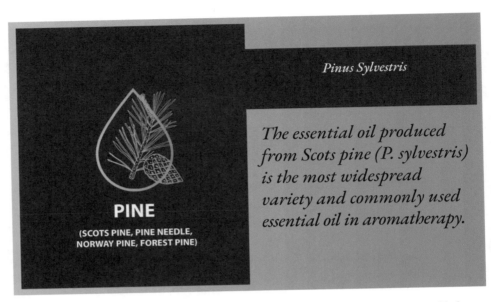

Pinus Sylvestris

PINE
(SCOTS PINE, PINE NEEDLE, NORWAY PINE, FOREST PINE)

The essential oil produced from Scots pine (P. sylvestris) is the most widespread variety and commonly used essential oil in aromatherapy.

Pine (Scots, Norway, Forest Pine & Pine Needle)
Pinus Sylvestris

Scots pine is a tree with leaves/needles in two-leaved fascicle (clusters); deep-fissured, reddish-brown bark that grows up to 40 meters high (131 feet tall). The Pinus genus consists of more than 100 species of coniferous trees, all producing a resin from which turpentine oil can be extracted. The Scots or Norway pine is the most widespread variety, as well as the safest and most useful therapeutically, though maritime pine (*Pinus pinaster*) and terebinth (Pinus mugo) are also important.

According to Salvatore Battaglia, the following are distinct types of pine essential oils:[169]

- Pine (Scots): *Pinus sylvestris L.*
- Pine (black): *Pinus nigra x JFArnold*
- Pine (dwarf): *Pinus mugo turra, Pinus mugo, Turra var. pumilio*
- Pine (white): *Pinus strobus L.*
- Pine (longleaf): *Pinus palustris*

While native to northern Europe and Russia, Scots pine grows abundantly in North America as well. The needles, young branches, and cones can all be used in the distillation process, although the best quality essential oil is extracted from the needles alone. The straight unbranched cylindrical trunks of the pine have furnished valuable timber for centuries and were once the favorite source of masts for sailing ships. The kernels were eaten by the ancient Egyptians, who added them to bread, while the young tops were used by the American Indians to prevent scurvy. They would also burn twigs along with cedar and juniper for ritual smudging of the sweat lodge to purify the spirit. Both the Swiss and Native Americans used the dried needles to stuff their mattresses, providing sweet smelling bedding that (inhibited) pests. Both Pidanius Dioscorides and Claudius Galen recommended ingesting the tree cones, especially when boiled with horehound and honey, to relieve a lingering cough and the cleansing of the chest and lungs. Traditional practice in Greece and Rome included adding the young, macerated shoots to a bath to relieve rheumatic pain and nervous tension. [170]

The best quality of *P. Sylvestris* pine oil comes from Tyrol, Australia. Pine essential oil is also obtained by steam distillation of the heartwood and stump wood of *P. Palustris* and other pinus species. This oil is then fractionally distilled under vacuum to yield pine oil. The lighter fractions from this distillate are known as wood turpentine. Production of this oil takes place mainly in the United States. Pine needle oil is extensively used in pharmaceutical preparations for cough and cold medicines, vaporizing fluids, nasal decongestants and analgesic ointments. [171]

According to Marcel Lavabre, the indications for this essential oil is for pulmonary diseases and urinary infections. [172] Kurt Schnaubelt suggests that pine oil, like other needle oils, has both anti-infectious and antifungal properties, and that its decongestant qualities for the upper respiratory tract are extremely effective. It is a forceful tonic and adrenal stimulant. Specifically, it can be used topically over the kidney area (10% in a base oil) for adrenal support and adrenals production, including adrenaline and prednisone, the body's natural cortisone. His preferred mode of use is the topical only. This essential oil should never be taken orally. He finds that the quality of commercially available pine essential oil is generally acceptable. [173]

1. **Class**: Monoterpenes

2. **Family**: *Pinaceae*

3. **Distillation**: *P. sylvestris* essential oil is steam distilled from the needles, young branches (twigs), and cones.

4. **Biochemical**:
   a. Monoterpenes (high %): (-) & (+)-α & (-)-β-pinene (>41 &<12%), limonene (up to 30%), -3-carene
   b. Sesquiterpenes: longifolene
   c. Alcohols: borneol (2.0%), α-cadinol, muurolols
   d. Esters: bornyl acetate (up to 10%)

5. **Uses**:
   a. Antimicrobial
   b. Antifungal
   c. Antiphlogistic
   d. Anti-infectious
   e. Antineuralgic
   f. Antirheumatic
   g. Antiscorbutic
   h. Antidiabetic (pituitary pancreatic axis)
   i. Antiseptic (pulmonary, urinary, hepatic)
   j. Antiviral
   k. Bactericidal (staph, pigmented, e. coli, proteus)
   l. Balsamic
   m. Cholagogue
   n. Choleretic
   o. Cortisone-like (pituitary-gonad sexual stimulant)
   p. Deodorant
   q. Decongestant (lymphatic, utero-ovarian)
   r. Diuretic
   s. Expectorant
   t. Hypertensive
   u. Hormone-like
   v. Insecticidal
   w. Nervous system
   x. Restorative
   y. Rubefacient
   z. Tonic (stimulant: adrenal cortex, circulatory)
   aa. Udorific
   ab. Vermifuge

VETERINARY USE: Excellent for bronchial afflictions, balsamic control is a treatment used on horses. It contains four ingredients (nigella, lemon, eucalyptus and garlic). Some horses are particularly sensitive to the quality of the air they breathe. The presence of dust, mold, or pollen can cause recurrent respiratory disorders or discomfort when the horse begins working, creating additional nutritional requirements. Such disorders can pose a problem to both horses and riders. It can also be used as an antiseptic, expectorant, and insecticide.

6. **Chemical composition:** Scots pine needle essential oil contains 50-97% monoterpene hydrocarbons composed mostly of α-pinene, with lesser amounts of 3-carene, dipentene, β-pinene, d-limonene, α terpinene, γ-terpinene, cis-B-ocimene, myrcene, camphene, sabinene and terpinolene. Other compounds present include:[175]
      a. borneol acetate – 3 – 3.5%
      b. borneol
      c. 1,8 cineol
      d. citral
      e. terpineol
      f. caryophyllene
      g. butyric acid
      h. valeric acid
      i. caproic acid
      j. isocaproic acid

7. **Systems:**
      a. Integumentary: Provides support for boils, cuts, fleas, excessive perspiration, sores, eczema, psoriasis, ringworm, scabies, lice, and congested skin. Affects dermis layer and purifies skin, especially grey, discolored, and oxygen-deprived skin (found in regular/chronic smokers)

b. Respiratory: Eases breathing and provides support for asthma, bronchitis, catarrh, whooping coughs, sinusitis, sore throat, and laryngitis. Clears sinuses. Stimulates and purifies respiratory tract and circulation. Increases secretion of mucus membrane of lungs, increasing the CO_2 discharge. Most effective application via inhalation.

c. Muscular/skeletal: Supports various joint/muscular aches and pains. Provides relief from rheumatoid arthritis, rheumatism, gout, and sciatica. Relieves edema (simple water retention) and stiffness. Provides support for multiple sclerosis.

d. Cardiovascular/lymphatic: Stimulates poor circulation.

e. Immune: Serves as an immune stimulant. Warms and cools fevers. Provides support for colds and flu. Modulates inflammatory and allergic processes. Aids severe infections.

f. Digestive: Provides support for intestinal disturbances, hepatitis, and inflamed gallbladder. Stimulates metabolism (pancreas) and provides support for diabetes.

g. Endocrine: Supports thyroid (caution here with thyroid imbalances). Stimulates adrenal (cortisone-like action). Stimulates pituitary gonads.

h. Genito-urinary/reproductive: Provides support for cystitis, urinary infection, and inflamed and congested uterus. Serves as a male stimulant and restorative for prostate problems causing impotence.

i. Central nervous system: Combats fatigue, nervous exhaustion, debility, and neuralgia. Provides support for stress related conditions, and adrenal cortex stimulant. Refreshes the tired mind, is cleansing, and provides healing for hopelessness, low self-esteem, lack of energy, weakness, and nervous depletion.

8. **Personality**: The pine personality would be upright, direct, and sometimes self-righteous. Pine personalities are the soft, gentle types who often go through life afraid to make a sound, or a mistake, and when they do, will always say it was their fault. This personality can be self-critical, full of guilt, and constantly apologizing for everything and everyone. [174] Pine essential oil has been described as a symbol of an uncompromising will to live, exhibiting endurance, strength, and a free spirit that refuses to confirm or live, in servitude. This oil awakens one's spirit and supports people who lack courage, perseverance, self-confidence, and patience. [175] The character for pine essential oil includes is acceptance, understanding, patience, and self-forgiveness. This oil encourages these positive attributes: humility, simplicity, forgiving, perseverance, trusting, direction, acceptance of love, tenacity, confident and exhilarated. Pine oil counteracts these negative attributes: regret, shame, guilt, self-criticism, worry, hyper-responsibility, non-confrontational, unworthiness, exhaustion, masochism, shamefulness, rejection, and inadequacy. [176]

9. **Safety**: Tested at low dose to be non-toxic and non-irritant, but with possible sensitization. It appears that pine oils high in −3-carene, or oils that are oxidized could contain more potent sensitizing agents, causing dermatitis and eczema-type reactions; therefore, pine oil for aromatherapy use should be fresh. Cross reaction possible to pine balsam, spruce, and Peru and Tolu balsam.

10. **Blending**: Top note.

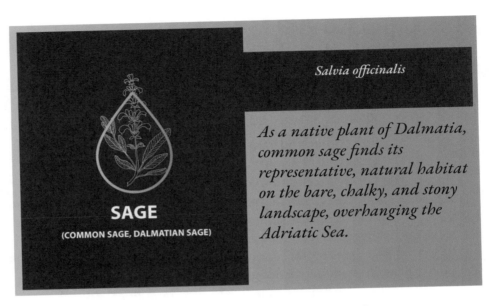

Salvia officinalis

As a native plant of Dalmatia, common sage finds its representative, natural habitat on the bare, chalky, and stony landscape, overhanging the Adriatic Sea.

Sage (Common Sage, Dalmatian Sage)
Salvia officinalis

Salvia officinalis, common sage is also known as true sage and has a history of use as a sacred herb and health-supporting tea in Europe, in Provence, and Greece, is one of those numerous so-called officinal plants and was used much by the apothecaries of the Middle Ages for making remedies. The plant was probably dispersed over the Alps into other areas of Europe by the travels of local monks. [177]

Salvia officinalis, the common sage or just sage, is a perennial, evergreen subshrub, with woody stems, grayish leaves, and blue to purplish flowers. It is a member of the mint family *Lamiaceae* and native to the Mediterranean region, though it has been naturalized in many places throughout the world.

According to Kurt Schnaubelt, sage oil has been shown to have an extremely broad spectrum of action in vitro. Because of its high content of ketone thujone, experiences regarding this oil are gathered slowly or not all. Published data supports the conclusion that whole/entire oil is less toxic than the thujone content would suggest. Sage essential oil is highly regenerative and because it dissolves lipids, it can be used to minimize cellulite. It is antibacterial, antifungal, and antiviral, and it mimics the action of estrogen in the body. His preferred mode of application is topical in skin care, and he recommends using it with caution in blends. He finds the quality of commercially available oils to vary. [178]

Marcel Lavabre states "It's been renowned since antiquity, the *salvia salvatrix* of the Romans is one of the most powerful and versatile medicinal plants Indeed, *Cur moriatur homo, cui slavia crescit in horto?* (Why should he die, the one who grows sage in his garden?) That panacea, which preserves health and youth was always recommended for conception and pregnancy." [179]

Robert Tisserand includes many different types of sage plants in his reference book "Essential Oil Safety, 2nd Edition" including:[180]

- ♣ Sage (African wild) *tarchonanthus camphoratus L. Asteraceae* family. Essential oil produced from leaves and flowers.
- ♣ Sage (Blue Mountain) *Salvia stenophylla Burch. Lamiaceae* family. Essential oil produced from leaves and stem.
- ♣ Sage (Dalmatian) *Salvia officinalis, Lamiaceae* family. Essential oil produced from leaves only.
- ♣ Sage (Greek) Turkish sage, *Salvia fruticosa Mill. Lamiaceae* family. Essential oil produced from leaves.
- ♣ Sage (Spanish) *Salvia lavandulifolia Vahl. Lamiaceae* family. Essential oil produced from flowering tops.
- ♣ Sage (White) *Salvia apiana Jeps. Lamiaceae* family. Essential oil produced from leaves.
- ♣ Sage (Wild Mountain) *Hemizygia petiolata Ashby. Lamiaceae* family. Essential oil produced from aerial parts above ground.

When ordering or using sage, each practitioner should understand which plant was used in the production of the essential oil and how the chemical constituents of the plant affect healing therapy. The detailed essential oil description provided below refers to the sage in the title, *Salvia officinalis.*

1. **Class**: Ketone, diterpenoid oxide

2. **Family**: *Lamiaceae* or *Labiatae* (also *Asteraceae* above)

3. **Distillation**: Steam distilled from the dried leaves

4. **Biochemical**:
   a. Monoterpenes: α-thujene, α-pinene, β-pinene, camphene, myrcene, α-terpinenes, limonene, cis & trans-ocimenes, allo-ocimene, paracymene, terpinolene

b.   Sesquiterpenes: β-caryophyllene, aromadendrene, allo-aromadendrene, α-humulene-4, D-cadinenes, β-copaene, α-corocalene, sellina-5,11-diene, ledene

c.   Hydrocarbons: cis-7-trans-2-methyl-3methyulene-hept-5-ane

d.   Alcohols: 1-octen-3-ol, linalool (>11%), terpinen-4-ol (4%), α-terpineol (5%) 8-terpinole, borneol, thujanol-4, p-cymenol-8, salviol

e.   Sesquiterpene alcohol: viridiflorol

f.   Esters: methyl isovalerate, bornyl, linalyl, sabinyl acetate: linalyl isovalerate

g.   Phenols: thymol

h.   Oxides: 1,8 cineol (up to 14%) Caryophyllene oxide

i.   Ketones: (approximately 60%): (-)-a-thujone (+)-B-thujone, camphor

j.   Coumarins: sesculetine

5.   **Uses:**

    a.   Anticellulite

    b.   Analgesic

    c.   Antibacterial (staphylococcus & streptococcus)

    d.   Anticancer (malignant conditions)

    e.   Anticatarrhal

    f.   Antifungal (candida albicans)

    g.   Anti-infectious

    h.   Anti-inflammatory

    i.   Antilactogenic

    j.   Antipyretic (hot flashes)

    k.   Antimicrobial

    l.   Antispasmodic

    m.   Antioxidant

    n.   Antiseptic

    o.   Astringent

    p.   Antisudorific

    q.   Antiviral

    r.   Cholagogue

s. Choleretic

t. Cicatrizant

u. Circulatory regulator

v. Depurative

w. Digestive

x. Diuretic

y. Drains biliary canal

z. Emmenagogic

aa. Estrogen-like

ab. Expectorant

ac. Hormone-like

ad. Febrifuge

ae. Hepatic

af. Hypertensive

ag. Hypoglycemia (pre-diabetes)

ah. Insecticidal

ai. Laxative

aj. Lipolytic

ak. Mucolytic

al. Neurotonic

6. **Chemical composition**: A typical chemical composition of sage essential oil produces from wild *S. officinalis* plants collected in Croatia in the month of June was reported as follows: [165]

a. α-pinene – 3.0%

b. camphene – 1.7%

c. β-pinene – 0.7%

d. limonene – 1.0%

e. 1,8 cineol – 13.2%

f. α-thujone – 23.1%

g. β-thujone – 25.0%

h. camphor - 9.5%

i. linalool – 0.5%

j. linalyl acetate – 0.8%

k. bornyl acetate – 0.9%

l. borneol – 1.4%

m. α-humulene – 1.2%

Sage is occasionally adulterated with other essential oils that have a similar odor profile such as cedar leaf (thuja) oil, Spanish sage, rosemary oil and various artemisia oils. The oil is also adulterated with β-caryophyllene, 1,8 cineol, and borneol from other sources. In turn, sage is also used an adulterant in other oils. The composition of *S. officinalis* essential oil is highly influenced by genetics and environmental factors such as season, climate conditions, and age of the plant when harvested. As a result, it does not always match the profile defined by ISO9909. [181]

7. **Systems**:
   a. Integumentary: Provides support for inflamed skin, oily secretions (skin and hair), dermatitis, psoriasis, skin ulcers, cold sores, radiation burns, herpes, shingles, insect bites, and edema (simple water retention). Provides supports for cuts and aids the formation of scar tissue. Supports regenerative skin care, constricts pores, and regulates excessive perspiration. Provides shine for hair, promotes hair growth, and reduces alopecia of hormonal origin.
   b. Respiratory: Increases resorption ability for mucus membranes or respiratory tract and sinuses. Aids coughs, catarrh, acute and chronic bronchitis, tuberculosis, asthma, colds, catarrh, flu, and sinusitis.
   c. Muscular/skeletal: Provides support for fibrositis (inflamed muscle), rheumatoid arthritis, painful muscles, and stiff neck, especially after sports. Eases trembling and palsy, elderly debility, sciatica, lumbago, and joint pain (rheumatoid and traumatic). Hydrates connective tissue.
   d. Cardiovascular/lymphatic: Raises low blood pressure, regulates circulation, arrests bleeding, aids varicosities; dissolves excess cholesterol, and aids lymphatic flow.

    e.   Immune: Serves as an immune stimulant, providing support for bacterial infections, colds, flu, and viral meningitis.

    f.   Digestive: Serves as a tonic to digestion, combats intestinal putrefaction, clears mucus from liver, stimulates gallbladder, increases cellular resorption in intestines, raises blood sugar level, decreases cholesterol levels, and aids elimination of toxins. Treats mouth ulcers and gingivitis. Provides energy to body. Stimulates and balances liver.

    g.   Endocrine: Promotes adrenal medulla hormones (adrenaline and nor-adrenaline) estrogen stimulant.

    h.   Genito-urinary/reproductive: Used as an herbal extract (internally), regulates menstrual cycle when it is scanty (similar to estrogen). Induces menstruation and pre-post-menopausal sweating. Aids vaginal thrush, leucorrhea, genital herpes, and condyloma. Regulates excretion and supports eliminations of toxins.

    i.   Central nervous system: Provides support for viral meningitis and viral neuritis. Eases depression, mental strain and exhaustion. At a low dose, calms PNS brain and motor nerves to relieve tiredness, depression, and grief. Quickens the senses, aids memory, brings wisdom, and clears negative energy from a room before meditation. Serves as an emotional purifier, eases rigidity.

8.   **Personality**: "*Salvia officinalis* evokes the huntress, Artemis, the lunar goddess and eternal virgin. A symbol of the feminine principle, of the soul of the world which the solar spirit, the creator Logos, brought forth from himself, Artemis, in his energy materialized, the matter in which he contemplates himself, in the life which animate and gives from to every earthbound create. 'You were

for a moment beside me, and you made me sense the great mystery of woman which beats in the very heart of Creation.' sang Rabindranath Tagore in homage to the eternal woman. Protector of women, children and wild animals and birth, Artemis saves her proteges, but like any lunar principle, she wears a double face and although she controls the art of healing as holding the might to protect her own, she also possesses the power to spread disease and bring death." [182] *Salvia officinalis* is a beautiful female oil. It will give a girl the basics of wisdom for her to cross over into womanhood and open her eyes to the risks she is running through her naivety and lack of determination. [183] Sage is an essence and a character needing to be discovered, and it can give a glimpse of wondrous nature when one has gotten past one's initial fear in the face of Cerberus, the guardian of the threshold who is sure to be there, with such a treasure. [184]

9. **Safety**: The essential oil of sage is toxic at high doses and should not be taken internally for extended periods of time. It is not recommended for people with epileptic tendencies. [185]

    Robert Tisserand's safety summary includes: [186]

    ♠ Hazards: neurotoxicity
    ♠ Contraindications: should not be taken in oral doses
    ♠ Contraindications (all routes): pregnancy, breastfeeding
    ♠ Maximum dermal use level: 0.4%

10. **Blending**: Top note.

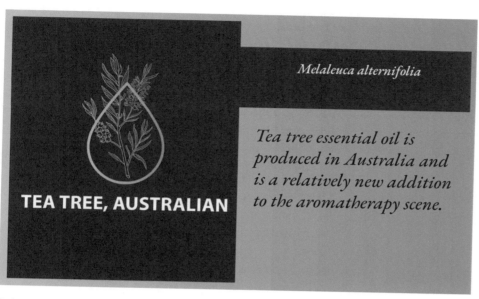

Melaleuca alternifolia

Tea tree essential oil is produced in Australia and is a relatively new addition to the aromatherapy scene.

Tea Tree, Australian
Melaleuca alternifolia

The oil has been accepted by many as a universal panacea and a welcome addition to the homeopathic first aid kit. Because of its properties, *Melaleuca alternifolia* is one of the most widely documented essential oils for its medical and antiseptic properties. *M. alternifolia* is a small tree with needle-type leaves (similar to cypress) that demonstrates amazing vitality. This tree grows in swampy, marshy areas and yields one of the best antifungals, anti-infectious, and antiseptic oils, indicating its strong immunostimulant properties. Before the demand for its oil increased dramatically in the 1980s, tea tree was considered a weed – a real plague – and farmers could not get rid of it. [187]

M. alternifolia grows between 5 and 7 meters tall, usually with a single trunk, but it may have multiple stems originating from common rootstock. Most of the oil available nowadays is from commercial plantations. The Australian aborigines have long recognized the virtues of tea tree. The leaves were simply crushed in the hand and the volatile oil inhaled to relieve colds and headaches. When the leaves were brewed into a tea, the drink was to prevent scurvy. Tea tree oil was first distilled for common use in Australia in 1920. [188]

Because the water-resistant "paperbark" is so easily peeled off the tree, it was used extensively by the aboriginal natives of Australia to make small canoes, knife sheaths, and thatching for shelters. According to the British Medical

Journal in 1933, tea tree became recognized as "a powerful disinfectant, non-poisonous and non-irritating." Indeed, among the essential oils valued for their anti-infectious properties, tea tree has few rivals. [189]

The aborigines have bark paintings of the "lightening god," which is reminiscent of the lightning-quick force of tea tree oil in combating infection and disease. [190] A 1962 American study of 130 women treated for vaginal infection and trichomoniasis using a tampon with tea tree essential oil found that all 130 recovered from the infection. without additional medical intervention. Tea tree oil may be added to a vaginal douche (5 drops in 4 ounces of water) or applied with a tampon treated with 5% tea tree salve. [191]

1.   **Class**: Monoterpenes, alcohol

2.   **Family**: *Myrtaceae*

3.   **Distillation**: Water or steamed distilled from the tea tree leaves

4.   **Biochemical**:
   a.   Monoterpenes: α-pinene, β-pinene, myrcene, α & y-terpenes, paracymene, limonene, terpinolene
   b.   Sesquiterpenes: β-caryophyllene, aromadendrene, allo-aromadendrene, viridiflorene, α & β-cadinene
   c.   Alcohols (approx. 50%): (+) terpinen-4-ol (>59%), α-terpineol, β-terpineol, para cymonol-8, cis & trans thujanol-4, globulol, viridiflorol
   d.   Oxides: 1,4 cineole, 1,8 cineol (>18% epoxy caryophyllene)

5.   **Uses**:
   a.   Antiasthenic
   b.   Anti-inflammatory
   c.   Antipruritic
   d.   Antiviral
   e.   Anti-infectious

f. Antimicrobial

g. Antifungal

h. Antiseptic

i. Bactericide (staphylococcus, e. coli, Krebs cycle disorders)

j. Balsamic

k. Cardiotonic (ventricular)

l. Cicatrizant

m. Cordial

n. Diaphoretic

o. Decongestant

p. Expectorant

q. Fungicide

r. Immunostimulant (immunoglobulin A [IgA] & immunoglobulin M [IgM])

s. Insecticide

t. Stimulant

u. Sudorific

6. **Chemical composition**: A typical chemical composition of tea tree is reported as follows: [188]

a. α-pinene – 2.1%

b. β-pinene – 0.4%

c. sabinene – 0.2%

d. myrcene – 0.4%

e. α-phellandrene – 0.8%

f. α-terpinene – 7.1%

g. limonene – 1.4%

h. 1,8 cineol – 3.0%

i. y-terpinene – 15.7%

j. para-cymene – 6.2%

k. terpinolene – 3.4%

l. linalool – 0.02%

m. terpinen-4-ol – 45.4%

n. α-terpineol – 5.3%

The Australian standard for tea tree oil (AS 2782, 1985) requires that 1,8 cineol content shall not exceed 15% and the terpinen-4-ol content shall be at least 30%. Research has been conducted to determine the microbiological activity of the essential oil with regards to the terpinen-4-ol to cineol ratio. However, maintaining quality control when harvesting from the bush creates challenges because the *M. alternifolia* tree may produce oil with cineol content ranting from 1 to 65%. [192]

7. **Systems**:

   a. Integumentary: Provides support for acne, abscess, athletes' foot, herpes, dandruff, oily skin, rashes, warts, diabetic gangrene, impetigo, ringworm, pediculosis, and wounds. Protects skin from burns during radiation treatments and after treatment when used in combination with rose and lavender.

   b. Respiratory: Provides support for asthma, bronchitis, and emphysema (with infection), catarrh, coughs, tuberculosis, sinusitis, and whooping cough. Also provides excellent support for tonsilitis, ear and nose and throat infections.

   c. Cardiovascular: Stimulates circulation within in the capillaries and cerebral. Aids with hemorrhoids, varicosities, and aneurysms, especially during medical emergencies. May also provide support in aftercare. Stimulates lymphatic circulation.

   d. Immune: Serves as an immune stimulant (IgA), especially for colds, flu, fever, streptococcus and staphylococcus infections. Supports body's response to viral and fungal infections including candida and children's infections such as chicken pox. Excellent preventative when used in combination with rosewood, thyme linalool, and ravensara. Provides support for shock before surgery used in combination with niaouli.

e.   Digestive: Provides support for mouth ulcers, gingivitis, oral mucosa inflammation, dental abscesses, oral ulcers, and pyorrhea. Excellent support for sore throats, bacteria, and parasites in digestive system. Provides protection from intestinal infections (2-3 drops in mineral water).

f.   Genito-urinary/reproductive: Provides excellent support for thrush, vaginitis, cystitis, pruritus, and all genital or reproductive system infections.

g.   Central nervous system: Serves as an energy stimulant and can be used for shock, asthenia, general and nervous exhaustion, and nervous depression.

8.   **Personality**: Tea tree's character fall under "leafies" personality. Their aspirations are to connect with the environment, understand global perspective, and gain wisdom. They are wise visionaries who know where they have come from and where our world in danger of going. Their minds are always alert, and they take in everything in an instant, and brake is down into its components parts and store it aware for future reference. Knowledge is their sustenance. They are not only extremely curious and knowledgeable, but also perceptive, intuitive, focused, insightful, and inspired. However, leafies may suffer intellectual delusions, almost as if reality were not important. They are vulnerable to criticism and can feel threatened by the slightest word. On a more personal level, the impoverish feels the unworthiness and although they are brilliant, they can be wrong sometimes and refuse to accept that they are wrong, they can become compulsive, ill-humored, scornful, and defeatist. The recluses are often impoverished "leafies", who already have a leaning towards secretiveness and isolation. They can become out of touch. [193]

9. **Safety**: Tea tree essential oil is non-toxic, non-irritant, and possibly sensitizing to some individuals. Researchers found that the tea tree oil that had been stored in clear glass bottles changed significantly from 3 to 30% of para-cymene in exposure to light. [194]
    According to Scylla Sheppard-Hanger, there is a possibility of skin irritation, and it has not been tested for sensitization at levels higher than 1% dilution. [195]

10. **Blending**: Top note.

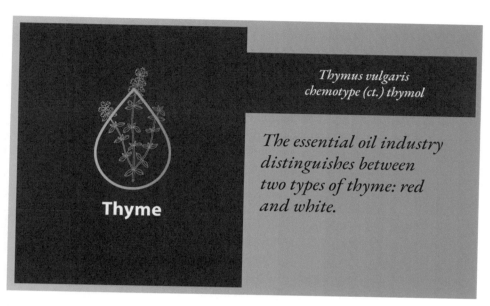

Thymus vulgaris chemotype (ct.) thymol

The essential oil industry distinguishes between two types of thyme: red and white.

Thyme, Red
Thymus vulgaris chemotype (ct.) thymol

There are more than 300 different varieties of thyme. White thyme is a rectified red thyme oil that is often compounded with pine oil, rosemary, and eucalyptus fractions.

There are six diverse types of chemotypes of *T. vulgaris*. Located close to the Mediterranean Sea at a low altitude, the two most common ones are the thymol type and the carvacrol type. The *Thymus vulgaris ct. linalool* prefers the sun and south-exposed slopes.

The most common types of *T. vulgaris* is known as garden or common thyme. Other species include *T. serpyllum*, known as creeping thyme or mother thyme; *T. zygis*, known as Spanish thyme; and *T. citrodorus* known as lemon thyme. In the Middle Ages, St. Hildegarde prescribed thyme for plague and paralysis, leprosy, and body lice. Thyme was included in the posies carried by judges and kings to protect them from disease in the public. Interestingly, thyme was used in combination with clove, lemon, and chamomile essential oils as a disinfectant and antiseptic in hospitals until World War I. The blend could kill yellow fever organisms and was seven times stronger than carbolic acid.[196]

Thymus vulgaris ct. thymol essential oil possesses qualities that are deep, long, lasting, consistent, and provide support for multiple challenges to the human body. The most common healing application is as an infection-fighting agent that is almost as powerful, but less violent and aggressive than *Satureja montana* (winter savory). Due to its low level of carvacrol, *Thymus vulgaris* ct. thymol acts deeply with the body's chemistry and restabilizes the terrain, particularly where repeated infectious pathologies occur. Used in combination with *Mentha piperita* (Peppermint) and *Daucus carota* (wild carrot essential oil), it fights debility and cleanses the gastro-intestinal area, especially when blended with *Rosmarinus officinalis* ct. bornyl acetate, verbenone blend with Lavandula spica for external treatment and diluted with vegetable oil. [197]

1. **Class**: Phenol

2. **Family**: *Lamiaceae* or *Labiatae*

3. **Distillation**: Produced by water and steam distillation of the dried or partially dried leaves and flowering tops of thyme

4. **Biochemical**:
   a. Monoterpenes and sesquiterpenes: paracymene, y-terpinene, pinene, camphene, β-caryophyllene
   b. Phenols: thymol, carvacrol
   c. Alcohols: high termpinen-4-ol, borneol, linalool, thuyanol, geraniol
   d. Esters: linalyl & bornyl acetate
   e. Esters: methyl thymol (trace), methyl carvacrol (trace)
   f. Oxide: cineol (trace)
   g. Ketone: camphor
   h. Citral: menthone
   (Also: triterpenic acids.)

5. **Uses**:
   a. Analgesic
   b. Anthelmintic
   c. Antimicrobial
   d. Antioxidant
   e. Antiputrefactive
   f. Antirheumatic

g. Antiseptic (intestinal pulmonary and urinary)
h. Antispasmodic
i. Anti-infectious (extremely powerful, large spectrum including anthrax, staph, e. coli, strep)
j. Antitussive
k. Antitoxic
l. Aperitif
m. Astringent
n. Aphrodisiac
o. Alsamic
p. Bechic
q. Bactericide
r. Cardiac
s. Carminative
t. Cicatrizant
u. Cholagogue
v. Choleretic
w. Diuretic
x. Digestive
y. Depurative
z. Emmenagogue
aa. Expectorant
ab. Euphoric
ac. Fungicidal
ad. Hypertensive
ae. Insecticide
af. Nervine
ag. Parasiticide
ah. Revulsive
ai. Rubefacient
aj. Stimulant (immune & circulatory)
ak. Tonic (general)
al. Vermifuge

Veterinary use: bronchitis, cicatrizant, parasiticide (scabies), gaseous indigestion (chronic ruminant, septicemic)

6. **Chemical composition**: A typical chemical composition of *T. vulgaris* and *T. zygis* is reported in the following table:

Constituent	*T. vulgaris*			*T.*
	ct. thymol	ct. carvacrol	ct. linalool	
α-thujone	4.6%	4.9%	0.26%	1.5
α-pinene	0.75%	4.3%	0.3%	0.7
camphene	0.3%	0.8%	0.27%	0.2
β-pinene	0.34%	0.35%	-	0.1
para-cymene	26%	33.9%	2.0%	25.
α-terpinene	24.0%	44.85%	0.28%	4.8
linalool	4.2%	4.2%	77.5%	3.4
borneol	0.65%	0.8%	0.2%	-
β-caryophyllene	3.55%	2.5%	2.85%	2.5
thymol	34.0%	5.5%	2.2%	8.3
carvacrol	4.7%	24.5%	trace	14.
geraniol	-	-	-	9.0

Battaglia, S. [198]

7. **Systems**:
   a. Integumentary – Caution, may be dangerous if applied as undiluted essential oil. Provides support for abscesses, insect bites, lice, scalp tonic, dandruff, and acne. Herbal extracts offer many more uses.
   b. Respiratory: Excellent support for asthma, spasms, bronchitis, pneumonia, colds, coughs, sore throat, and whooping cough. Supports the body's fight against flu and bronchitis, especially via inhalation used in combination with eucalyptus, cypress, niaouli and others. Purifies, clears, and detoxifies lungs and mucus membrane including sinuses. Excellent air antiseptic.

c. Muscular/skeletal: Provides support for arthritis, sciatica, rheumatism, gout pain, muscular aches and pains, and sprains especially for swelling, inflammation, and sports injuries. Combats asthenia, releases blocked joints, restores mobility, and aids rheumatism and arthritis.

d. Cardiovascular/lymphatic: Supports poor circulation and raises low blood pressure.

e. Immune: Excellent support for all infectious diseases. Stimulates white blood cells to combat infectious pathology. Serves as one of the most antiseptic essential oils for disinfecting air. Treats fragile terrain after serious infections.

f. Digestive: Stimulates sluggish digestion. Provides support for intestinal infection, antiseptic, upset stomach, and toxic headache. Purifies and clears mucus, detoxifies intestines, and treats intestinal parasites: ancylostoma, ascaris, and oxyurids.

g. Endocrine: Serves as an adrenal cortex stimulant (corticosteroid). Stimulates metabolism and sex hormones.

h. Genito-urinary/reproductive: Serves as a diuretic because of irritancy. Aids gout, edema from simple water retention. Serves as a urinary antiseptic, induces menstruation, and aids leucorrhea. Purifies and clears mucus and detoxifies urinary system including kidney, bladder, urinary tract, urinary duct, urethra, and uterus.

i. Central nervous system: Combats general fatigue, depression, and insomnia. Strengthens nerves, aids memory and concentration. Elevates low spirits and may help release mental blocks from trauma. Releases exhaustion; gives courage and emotional lift. Calms and relaxes anger and frustration

8. **Personality**: According to Mailhebiau, the thyme character is of a man of the soil, solid and squat, tanned skin and leathered complexion, the smile of simplicity and kindness lights up his face, which is burned by the sun and etched by the furrows of age. This essential oil carries about him the mark of his laborious life – simple, prosaic, but truthful. Not much given to speaking, he experiences things more than he rationalizes them, then only rarely and discreetly reveals what he experiences. His intelligence is intuitive, his knowledge spontaneous, and his kindness natural and modest. This character lives with a clear and wholesome spirit, devoid of sterile intellectualism, in tune with the rhythm of the earth and its seasons, must therefore resolve – at the risk of otherwise falling asleep forever – to gain a foothold in socio-cultural advancement, even if it means giving up a part of his wild and autarkical experience. Love of the earth demands that he should firstly take proper care of his own earth – the physical body – his needs being those of a particular time, the present, albeit imperfect and often incomprehensible. [199]

9. **Safety**: Tested at low level to be non-toxic, highly irritant, non-sensitizing. Not for use on damaged or sensitive skin. Inhalations may be preferred over massage and bath. Avoid with pregnancy or high blood pressure. Hepatotoxic in large amount and prolonged use.

10. **Blending**: Top/Middle note.

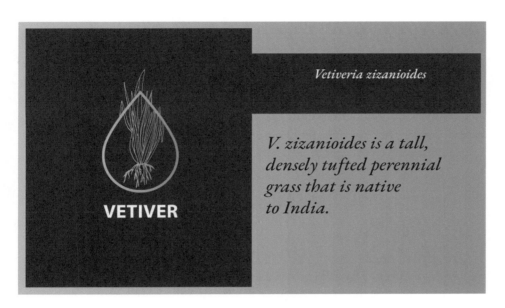

Vetiveria zizanioides

V. zizanioides is a tall, densely tufted perennial grass that is native to India.

Vetiver
Vetiveria zizanioides

The main root stack is a stout, branching rhizome developing an extensive but not deeply penetrating fibrous mat of aromatic roots. Most Indian, Sri Lankan, and Malaysian oil is produced from wild plants. Vetiver is grown commercially for oil in Java, the Seychelles, Reunion, Brazil, Haiti, and Japan. In India, oil produced from vetiver collected in the wild, and cultivated vetiver is differentiated by calling the former khus oil and the latter vetiver oil. The finest quality vetiver is referred to as bourbon vetiver and originates from the Reunion islands [200]

According to Kurt Schnaubelt, vetiver oil is a powerful circulatory and immunostimulant. Receptor processes explaining vetiver's action on the circulatory system could be recently demonstrated in controlled experiments. Vetiver has a warm earthy fragrance that can strike an intimate chord with many individuals. His preferred mode of use is topically and in fragrance compositions. He finds that the most reliable qualities seem to come from Central America. [201]

The *Gramineae* family produce the most sacred foods of the vegetable kingdom: wheat, rice, and corn—food beyond food, gift of the gods to the human realm. Vetiver expresses this fundamental aspect of the type through its sandalwood-like note, it is inspiring and uplifting. [202]

Vetiver's ability to cool and nourish the body is reflected in its actions on a psychological level. Relaxing an overheated, hyperactive mind and nurturing an insecure self-identity, the oil imbues the calm reassuring strength of mother earth, and her deep sense of belonging. Whether mentally exhausted from overwork, or out of touch with the physical body and its needs, vetiver sedates and yet restores – centers and reconnects – closing the gap between spirit and matter. According to the Indian philosophy of Vedanta, Prakriti is a feminine symbol of universal energy and of the power of manifestation. Through its capacity to reconnect us to our vital source, vetiver oil instils a sense of her potency [203]

1. **Class**: Alcohol, ketone

2. **Family**: *Gramineae*

3. **Distillation**: Steam distilled from cleaned and washed rootlets which are dried, cut and chopped, then soaked in water before distillation.

4. **Biochemical**:
   a. Sesquiterpenes: vetivene, tricyclovetivene, vetivazulene
   b. Sesquiterpenols: vetiverol, tricyclovetivenol, zizanol, furfurol
   c. Esters: vetiveryl acetate, benzoic acid
   d. Ketones: α- & β-vetivones

5. **Uses**:
   a. Antiseptic
   b. Antispasmodic
   c. Aphrodisiac
   d. Cytophylactic
   e. Circulatory and red corpuscles stimulant
   f. Depurative
   g. Emmenagogue
   h. Immune stimulant
   i. Nervine
   j. Sedative
   k. Rubefacient (mild)
   l. Tonic (glandular)
   m. Vermifuge

6. **Chemical composition**: The chemical composition of vetiver is considered complex. The main constituent in vetiver is vetiverol occurring between 50 to 75%. Three carbonyl compounds, α-vetivone, β-vetivone, and khusimone are considered to be the primary odor-influencing constituents. [200]

7. **Systems**:
   a. Integumentary: Provides support for acne, cuts, irritated wounds, urticaria, infections and inflammations. As a cell regenerator, provides excellent support for dry, mature skin as well as oily skin. Eases masculine aging signs for character. Works on dermis layer to correct astrophic and slack skin. Increases adipose base. Softens, hydrates, and detoxifies connective tissue.
   b. Muscular/skeletal: Provides support for arthritis, muscle aches, pains, and sprains including stiffness, rheumatism, and connective tissue challenges. Circulation stimulant that increases entire venous vessel system to activate blood supply and/or to detoxify connective tissue.
   c. Cardiovascular/lymphatic: Fortifies red blood cells while increasing oxygen. Stimulates circulation including arterial venous and is vasodilating. Activates venous circulation of lymphatic system.
   d. Immune: Cool fevers. Stimulates and aids depressed immune system.
   e. Digestive: Activates venous circulation in digestive organs epithelia cells including lymphatic vessels. May stimulate the pancreas and aid liver congestion.
   f. Endocrine: Pancreatic stimulate that may provide support for diabetes.

g. Genito-urinary/reproductive: Tonic to urinary excreting system. Stimulates cells' resorptive power. Aids impotence and frigidity. Induces menstruation when scanty and sluggish. Eases post-partum depression.

h. Central nervous system: Supports debility, depression, insomnia, nervous tension, mental and physical exhaustion. Balances central nervous system, grounds thoughts, and eases tranquilizers. Stimulates mind for more vitality, cleans aura, and strengthens auric shield.

8. **Personality**: According to Worwood, vetivers are often strong and intellectual with a strong sense of reality and awareness of what is happening around them, embodying the relationship between mind and body. Although the fragrance is often associated with the masculine, the vetiver personality, whether male or female, will be perfectly balanced between their masculine and feminine sides. There is nothing delicate or ethereal about the Vetiver profile. It's very much of the here and now. [204]

Vetiver oil connects us to the earth's energies. It is a source of vital energy and generation. The earthy fragrance of the oil supports all those who have lost touch with the earth or with their roots. Vetiver nourishes people who have cold feet or have their heads in the clouds. When we lose contact with the ground beneath us, with reality, we pay the price of a weakened immune system. When in touch with the earth, we breathe fresh air, enjoy the magic of an open fire, and feel the wind blow through our hair. [205]

When turning points of life bring a challenge to face its shadows, vetiver, with its stabilizing tranquility, brings a quiet assurance, drawing you to the earth, offering support and strength as you reconcile the changes taking place. If you are feeling threatened by the demands of your own soul for change, vetiver will embrace, sustain, and re-establish a balanced relationship between your heart, body, and mind [206]

9. **Safety**: Tested at low dose, non-toxic, non-irritant and non-sensitizing; rare report of dermatitis in hypertensive individuals.

10. **Blending**: Base note.

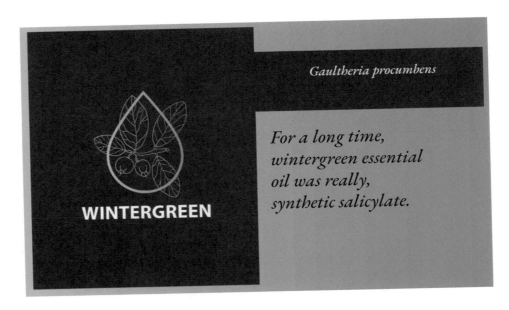

Gaultheria procumbens

For a long time, wintergreen essential oil was really, synthetic salicylate.

Wintergreen
Gaultheria procumbens

For a number of years now, true distilled oil is again available from Nepal, distilled not from *Gaultheria procumbens*, as in North America, but from *Gaultheria fragrantissima*. The oil is traditionally used for its anti-inflammative and analgesic effect. It can be mediated by a process known as counterirritation for rheumatoid arthritis. The oil is a strong irritant if used in high concentration. It should always be blended with other essential oils. Caution should be exercised in any application of this essential oil and ensuring its use via an extremely diluted blend. Dr. Schnaubelt's preferred mode of use is external only. As for the quality, it will be either genuine or synthetic. [207] Interestingly, Marcel Lavabre states that wintergreen essential oil is similar to birch oil in its composition; however, that oil is no longer produced. Therefore, all essential oil products sold as wintergreen are either methyl salicylate or birch oil. Food for thought! [208] Wintergreen oil is recommended for external application as a liniment because of its anti-inflammatory and antirheumatic properties, specifically for rheumatoid arthritis. Salicylates have the ability to suppress the synthesis of prostaglandins, which have an integral role in the management of pain and inflammation. [209])

When heavy with inertia and missing internal motivation, wintergreen, with its vigorous, strengthening action, will push you toward greater productivity, refocus your goals, and keep you on track. [210]

1. **Class**: Esters

2. **Family**: *Ericaceae*

3. **Distillation**: Wintergreen essential oil is derived by water distillation of the of *Gaultheria procumbens*. Prior to distillation, the leaves are exposed to enzymatic action in warm water. During this process, methyl salicylate is formed as a decomposition product from a glycoside in the plant material [209]. Rare true wintergreen is available that has not been adulterated with birch and/or red color. Wintergreen oil is a pale yellow to yellow-pink color with an intense sweet aroma. If it has been adulterated it will be red in color, which indicates iron impurities.

4. **Biochemical**:
    a. Methyl salicylate (Up to 99%)
        Also: triacontane and various aldehydes, ketones, and alcohols

5. **Uses**:
    a. Antiseptic
    b. Analgesic
    c. Antispasmodic
    d. Anti-inflammatory
    e. Antirheumatic
    f. Antitussive
    g. Astringent
    h. Carminative
    i. Diuretic
    j. Emmenagogue
    k. Hepato-stimulant
    l. Galactagogue
    m. Stimulant
    n. Vasodilator
    o. Vulnerary

6. **Chemical composition**: The main constituent found in wintergreen oils is methyl salicylate (98%). Most

commercial wintergreen essential oils contain only synthetic methyl salicylate. [211]

7. **Systems**:
   a. Integumentary: Provides support for eczema, acne, blemishes, and inflammation. Aids wounds and skin infections.
   b. Muscular/skeletal: Provides relief from sore muscles and works especially well blended with lavender, eucalyptus, peppermint, and camphor. Provides support for arthritis, rheumatoid epicondylitis, rheumatism, tendinitis, cramps, sprains, and sciatica.
   c. Cardiovascular/lymphatic: Provides support for coronaritis (crisis curative). Aids hypertension, arteriosclerosis, and lymphatic drainage.
   d. Digestive: Stimulates liver. Aids headache (especially hepato-circulatory origin). May provide support for diarrhea.
   e. Genito-urinary/reproductive: Aids nephritic colic. Provides relief from edema (simple water retention) and cellulite.
   f. Central nervous system: Provides support for headaches from liver congestion.

8. **Personality**: Since Wintergreen is distilled from leaves, it falls into the category of "leafies." Worwood states: *"They want to connect with the environment, understand the global perspective, and gain widespan wisdom."* Lateral thinking is a standard procedure for this type of person, as is looking at things holistically. Because they are innovative thinking, they often inventors, they are quite likely to have several original theories kicking around at the same time. These are profoundly creative people, intellectually, and they have an ingenious, original approach. No research lab should be without one.

9. **Safety**: Tisserand states that wintergreen oil is considered toxic and should not be used in aromatherapy. [213] However, the British Herbal Pharmacopeia recommends using wintergreen externally as a liniment. [214]

Tisserand also states high hazards with drug interaction, inhibits blood clotting, and toxicity (high doses are teratogenic). All application routes have contraindications, including anticoagulant mediation, major surgery, hemophilia, and other bleeding disorders. Also contraindicated for pregnancy, breastfeeding, children and people with salicylate sensitivity (often applied to ADD/ADHD). Also considered oral contraindication for gastroesophageal reflux disease (GERD) [215]

Caution: this oil is sensitive to damaged skin and should only be used locally when highly diluted (if at all). Tested to be hazardous. Moderately toxic. Irritant and sensitizing. Avoid in pregnancy, with babies, and for children.

10. **Blending**: Top note.

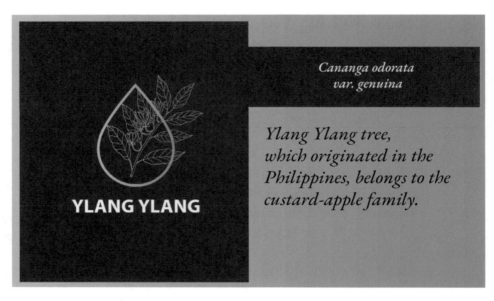

Cananga odorata
var. genuina

Ylang Ylang tree,
which originated in the
Philippines, belongs to the
custard-apple family.

Ylang Ylang
Cananga odorata var. genuina

Ylang Ylang is known as extra or bourbon, from the first distillation. Today, it is also cultivated in Java, Sumatra, Comoro Islands', Madagascar, Zanzibar, and Haiti. The tree grows to 66 feet with branches that bend slightly downward. The blossoms are unusually large, yellowish white, and have an intensely sweet scent. [216]

Because they bear seeds, all the plants used to obtain essential oils belong to the Spermatophyta subdivision. [217]According to the Prices, this beautiful oil has been suggested as a possible substitute for quinine in malaria and is a wonderful stimulant when applied as a mask or spraying. They mentioned that ylang ylang has been an old remedy for asthma, boils, diarrhea, head, malaria, ophthalmia, rheumatism, and stomach ailments. [218]

The aphrodisiac power of Ylang Ylang essential oil is inseparable both from its ability to relax ad uplift, and from its voluptuous aroma. Indicated for impotence and frigidity, it may be used by people whose fear, anxiety, and urge to withdraw have subconsciously blocked their feelings of sexuality. The love of the Hindu god Krishna for the milkmaid Radha symbolizes not only the union of masculine and feminine but of spirit and matter. [219]

According to Battaglia, Ylang Ylang essential oil is reported to exhibit good antibacterial properties against staph aureus. It was found to be one of the most popular choices of essential oils in a clinical trial using essential oils to control epileptic seizures. [220]

Distillation is carried out in small stills since the flowers would suffer considerably by the weight and pressure of a heavy charge of flowers. While the name suggests that the oil should be the natural distillate from the uninterrupted water and steam distillation, the complete blend is made by combining ylang ylang extra, first grade, and second grade fractions. The fractions are usually separated by controlling the specific gravity of the distillate. By controlling the specific gravity, producers make the interruptions at the moment when they feel that the oil can be classified within one of the groups. [221]

There are three grades of Ylang Ylang:
- ♠ Ylang Ylang extra is a pale yellow with a powerful floral and intensely sweet odor. The base note becomes more pleasant, softer, and sweeter.
- ♠ Ylang Ylang complete (made by combining oils) is usually a yellowish, somewhat- oily liquid with a powerful and intensely sweet but soft balsamic floral odor with a floral wood undertone.
- ♠ Ylang Ylang third grade is yellowish only liquid with a sweet floral odor and balsamic-woody base note

According to Sheppard-Hanger, the type available as "extra" is the top grade produced during the first hour, and then grades 1, 2, 3, are further distillates. They are also produced by concrete and absolute distillation.

1. **Class**: Esters

2. **Family**: *Annonaceae* (this family consists of one species, Cananga odorata)

3. **Distillation**: Steam distilled in small fractions from the flowers

4. **Biochemical**:
   a. Monoterpenes and sesquiterpenes: α-farnesene, pinene, cadinene
   b. Alcohols: (+)-linalool (up to 55%), benzyl acetate, farnesol, geraniol

c. Esters: geranyl acetate (>5%), benzyl acetate (10%), benzyl benzoate, linalyl acetate

d. Phenols: p-cresol, eugenol, isoeugenol

5. **Uses**:
   a. Aphrodisiac
   b. Antidepressant
   c. Antidiabetic
   d. Antiseptic
   e. Antispasmodic
   f. Euphoric
   g. Hypotensive
   h. Sedative (nervous nature)
   i. Stimulant (adrenal and circulatory)
   j. Tonic (general)

6. **Chemical composition**: Typical chemical composition of the various grades of ylang ylang are reported as follows:

Constituents	Extra (or bourbon)	1st grade (2nd distillation)	2nd grade (3rd distillation)	3rd grade (4th distillation)
linalool	13.6%	18.6%	2.8%	1.0%
geranyl acetate	5.3%	5.9%	4.1%	3.5%
caryophyllene	1.7%	6.0%	7.5%	9.0%
p-cresyl methyl ether	16.5%	7.6%	1.8%	0.5%
methyl benzoate	8.7%	6.4%	2.3%	1.0%
benzyl benzoate	2.2%	5.3%	4.7%	4.3%
other sesquiterpenes	7.4%	28.8%	54.5%	97.0%

Battaglia, S.[221]

7. **Systems**:
   a. Integumentary: Balances sebum. Aids irritated, dry, oily, and combination skin. Supports healing from acne. Serves as a general hair/skin

tonic for dry scalp. Promotes hair growth.
Provides relief from insect bites.

   b.   Respiratory: Slows breathing (hyperpnea).

   c.   Cardiovascular/lymphatic: Provides support for palpitations and tachycardia. Lowers blood pressure.

   d.   Immune: Provides support for fever, malaria, and typhoid.

   e.   Digestive: Aids diabetes. Balances and aids intestinal infections, diarrhea, and putrid fermentations.

   f.   Endocrine: Balances hormones, stimulates thymus gland, and regulates adrenal flow.

   g.   Genito-urinary/reproductive: Provides support for impotence and frigidity. Acts as an aphrodisiac. Serves as a uterus tonic and firms breast tissue.

   h.   Central nervous system: Provides support for depression, insomnia, nervous tension, stress-related pain, fear, rage, inner coldness, anger, low self-esteem, shock, and panic. Acts as a relaxant to the central nervous system.

8.   **Personality**: The Ylang Ylang personality is intensely feminine. She has a passionate nature, tempered by a calm and balance many find unnerving. Ylang ylang are people who delight in the erotic and sensual. No shrinking violets here! [222]

When you are angry, and volatile as a storm cloud, the striking intensity of Ylang Ylang matches the energy bound within. This exotic, sweet "flower of flowers" softens attitudes, breaks old patterns, and evokes flexibility. [223]

The spirit of ylang ylang usually fits the person naturally drawn to it. Upon inhaling ylang ylang with its heavy seductive, sweet aroma, one can imagine a fiery temperamental, passional and erotic person with an awesome radiance and confidence never losing her balance. She would also dress in bright and colorful clothing and loves to wear jewelry. The Ylang Ylang person is extremely passionate and feminine, charismatic, erotic, and sensual. Male or female, Ylang Ylang personalities are not happy alone, flourishing best when they have an audience to applaud their achievement. [217]

9. **Safety**: Tested at low dose, non-toxic, and non-irritant, possible sensitization; dermatitis reported in sensitized people. Do not use on inflamed skin or dermatitis conditions. Excess may lead to nausea and headache.

10. **Blending**: Middle/Base note.

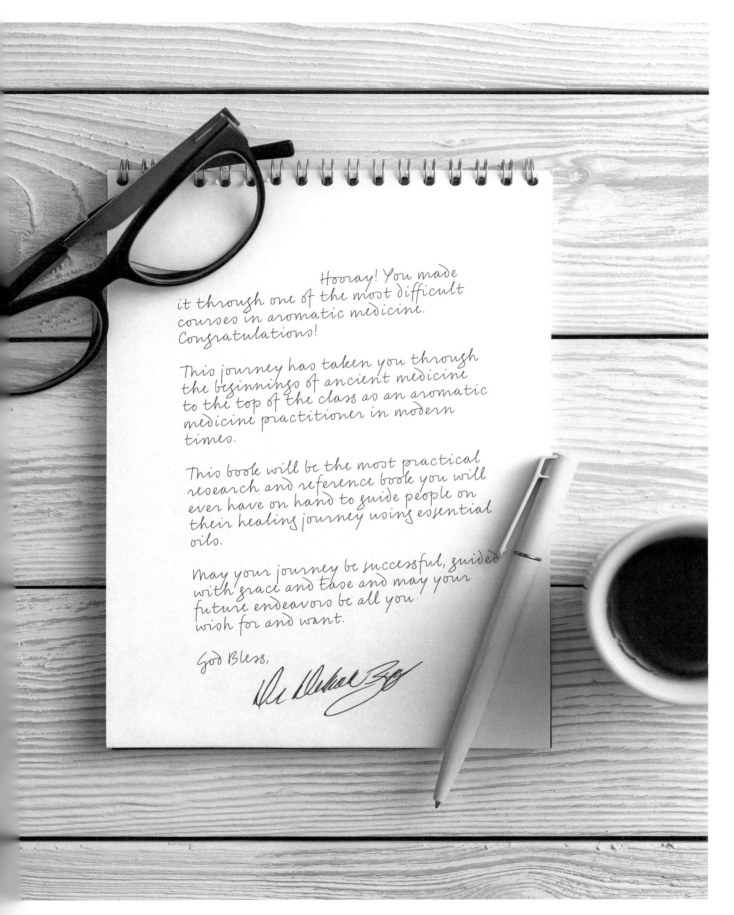

Hooray! You made it through one of the most difficult courses in aromatic medicine. Congratulations!

This journey has taken you through the beginnings of ancient medicine to the top of the class as an aromatic medicine practitioner in modern times.

This book will be the most practical research and reference book you will ever have on hand to guide people on their healing journey using essential oils.

May your journey be successful, guided with grace and ease and may your future endeavors be all you wish for and want.

God Bless,

Dr. Debra Bee

Chapter Sixteen References:

[1] Battaglia, S., *The Complete Guide to Aromatherapy, Volume III* - Psyche & Subtle, Black Pepper Creative Pty LTD, page 3.

[2] Battaglia, S., *The Complete Guide to Aromatherapy*, Perfect Potion Publisher, page 161.

[3] Fischer-Rizzi, S., *Complete Aromatherapy Handbook*, Sterling Publishing Co, page 60.

[4] Fischer-Rizzi, S., *Complete Aromatherapy Handbook*, Sterling Publishing Co, page 61.

[5] Battaglia, S., *The Complete Guide to Aromatherapy*, Perfect Potion Publisher, page 161.

[6] Battaglia, S., *The Complete Guide to Aromatherapy*, Perfect Potion Publisher, page 162.

[7] Battaglia, S., *The Complete Guide to Aromatherapy*, Perfect Potion Publisher, page 161.

[8] Sheppard-Hanger, S., *The Aromatherapy Practitioner Reference, Volume I, A-L,* The Atlantic Institute of Aromatherapy, page 107.

[9] Fischer-Rizzi, S., *Complete Aromatherapy Handbook*, S. Sterling Publishing Co, page 60.

[10] Leung, A. and Foster, S., *Encyclopedia of Common Natural Ingredients used in Foods, Drugs and Cosmetics, 2nd Ed.*, page 74.

[11] Schnaubelt, K., *Medical Aromatherapy: Healing with Essential Oils,* Frog Books, page 33 & 34.

[12] Worwood, V.A., *The Complete Book of Essential Oils,* New World Library, Page 569.

[13] Battaglia, S., *The Complete Guide to Aromatherapy, 2nd Ed.,* Perfect Potion Publisher, page 165.

[14] Worwood, V.A., *The Fragrant Mind,* New World Library, page 279.

[15] Battaglia, S.A., *The Complete Guide to Aromatherapy,* Perfect Potion Publisher, page 169.

[16] Worwood, V.A., *The Complete Book of Essential Oils,* New World Library, page 571.

[17] Tisserand, R. and Young R., *Essential Oil Safety,* 2nd Ed., Churchill Livingstone, page 508.

[18] Worwood, V.A. *The Fragrant Mind,* New World Library, page 283.

[19] Worwood, V.A., *The Fragrant Mind,* New World Library, page 218.

[20] Tisserand, R. and Balacs, T., *Essential Oil Safety,* Churchill Livingstone, page 121.

[21] Johnson S.A., *Evidence Based Essential Oil Therapy,* Create Space Independent Publishing Platform, July 11, 2015, page 59.

[22] Weiss, E.A., *Essential Oil Crops,* CAB international UK 1997, page 368.

[23] Battaglia, S., *The Complete Guide to Aromatherapy*, Perfect Potion Publisher, Page 171.

[24] Worwood, V.A., *The Complete Book of Essential Oils*, New World Library, page 283.

[25] Battaglia, S., *The Complete Guide to Aromatherapy*, Perfect Potion Publisher, page 184.

[26] Leung, A., Foster S., *Encyclopedia of Common Natural Ingredients used in Food, Drugs and Cosmetics, 2nd Ed.*, Wiley-Interscience, page 169.

[27] Leung, A, Foster S., *Encyclopedia of Common Natural Ingredients used in Food, Drugs and Cosmetics, 2nd Ed.*, Wiley-Interscience, page 168.

[28] Singh, H. B., et al., *"Cinnamon bark oil, a potent fungi-toxicant against fungi causing respiratory tract mycoses."* Allergy 1995: 50(12): 995-999 - cited in the Aromatherapy Database, Bob Harris, Essential oil Resource Consultants UK2000.

[29] Schnaubelt, K., *Medical Aromatherapy: Healing With Essential Oils*, Frog Books, page 215.

[30] Sheppard-Hanger, S., *The Aromatherapy Practitioner Reference Manual Volume I – A-L,* Atlantic Institute of Aromatherapy, 1995, page 157.

[31] Battaglia, S., *The Complete Guide to Aromatherapy,* Perfect Potion Publisher, page 185.

[32] Worwood, V.A., *The Complete Book of Essential Oils,* New World Library, page 295.

[33] Schnaubelt, K., *Medical Aromatherapy: Healing With Essential Oils,* Frog Books, page 174.

[34] Weiss, E.A., *Essential Oil Crops,* CAB international UK, 1997, page 6.

[35] Weiss, E.A., *Essential Oil Crops,* CAB international UK, 1997, page 235.

[36] Battaglia, S., *The Complete Guide to Aromatherapy, 2nd Ed*, Perfect Potion Publishing, page 190.

[37] Schnaubelt, K., *Medical Aromatherapy: Healing With Essential Oils,* Frog Books, pages 215-216

[38] Battaglia, S., *The Complete Guide to Aromatherapy, 2nd Ed*, Perfect Potion Publishing, page 191.

[39] Worwood, V.A., *The Fragrant Mind,* New World Library, page 227.

[40] Worwood, V.A., *The Fragrant Mind,* New World Library, page 231.

[41] Hartnoll, G., et al, *Near Fatal Ingestion of Oil of Clove,* Archive of Diseases in Childhood, 1993, page 392-393.

[42] Mailhebiau, P., *Portraits in Oil*s, C.W. Daniel publishing, page 49.

[43] Schnaubelt, K., *Medical Aromatherapy: Healing With Essential Oils*, Frog Books, page 38.

[44] Schnaubelt, K., *Medical Aromatherapy: Healing With Essential Oils*, Frog Books, page 182.

[45] Schnaubelt, K., *Medical Aromatherapy: Healing With Essential Oils*, Frog Books, page 211.

[46] Worwood, V.A., *The Fragrant Mind,* New World Library, page 302.

[47] Worwood, V.A., *The Fragrant Mind,* New World Library, page 303.

[48] Mailhebiau, P., *Portraits in Oils,* C.W. Daniel publishing. page 52.

[49] Schnaubelt, K., *Medical Aromatherapy: Healing With Essential Oils*, Frog Books, page 210.

[50] Battaglia, S., *The Complete Guide to Aromatherapy 2nd Ed*, Perfect Potion Publisher, page 199.

[51] Battaglia, S., *The Complete Guide to Aromatherapy, 2nd Ed,* Perfect Potion Publisher, page 199.

[52] Worwood, V.A., *The Fragrant Mind,* New World Library, page 318.

[53] Battaglia, S., *The Complete Guide to Aromatherapy, 2nd Ed,* Perfect Potion Publisher, page 206.

[54] Weiss, W.A., *Essential Oil Crops,*1997, CAB international, page 50.

[55] Lis-Balchin, M., *Geranium Oil: International Journal of Aromatherapy,* 1996, page 18.

[56] Battaglia, S., *The Complete Guide to Aromatherapy , 2nd Ed,* Perfect Potion Publisher, page 207.

[57] Worwood, V.A., *The Fragrant Mind, New World Library,* page 313.

[58] Worwood, V.A., *The Fragrant Mind,* New World Library, page 312.

[59] Price, S. & L., *Aromatherapy for Professionals, 3rd Ed,* Churchill Livingstone, page 450.

[60] Schnaubelt, K., *Medical Aromatherapy: Healing With Essentials Oils,* Frog Books, page 166.

[61] Schnaubelt, K., *Medical Aromatherapy: Healing With Essentials Oils,* Frog Books, page 209.

[62] Sheppard-Hanger, S., *The Aromatherapy Practitioner Reference Manual,* Volume II, Atlantic Institute of Aromatherapy, Page 275.

[63] Battaglia, S., *The Complete Guide to Aromatherapy,* Perfect Potion Publishing, page 180.

[64] Sheppard-Hanger, S., *The Aromatherapy Practitioner Reference Manual,* Volume II, M-Z, Atlantic Institute of Aromatherapy 1995, page 275.

[65] Battaglia, S., *The Complete Guide to Aromatherapy,* Perfect Potion Publishing, page 180.

[66] Worwood, V.A., *The Fragrant Mind,* New World Library, page 292.

[67] Battaglia, S., *The Complete Guide to Aromatherapy 2nd Ed,* Perfect Potion Publisher, page 210.

[68] Price, S. & L., *Aromatherapy for Professionals, 3rd Ed,* Churchill Livingstone, page 237.

[69] Schnaubelt, K., *Medical Aromatherapy: Healing with Essential Oils,* Frog Books, page 185.

[70] Worwood, V.A., *The Fragrant Mind,* New World Library, page 316.

[71] Schnaubelt, K., *Medical Aromatherapy: Healing with Essential Oils,* Frog Books, page 185.

[72] Price, S. & L., *Aromatherapy for Professionals, 3rd Ed,* Churchill Livingstone, page 408.

[73] Franchomme, P., & Penoel, D., *Home Health Care,* 2001, page 368.

[74] Sheppard-Hanger, S., *The Aromatherapy Practitioner Reference, Volume I – A-L.,* Atlantic Institute of Aromatherapy 1995, page 175.

[75] Battaglia, S., *The Complete Guide to Aromatherapy,* Perfect Potion Publisher, page 215.

[76] Worwood, V.A., *The Fragrant Mind,* New World Library, page 324.

[77] Battaglia, S., *The Complete Guide to Aromatherapy, 2nd Ed,* Perfect Potion Publisher, page 216.

[78] Battaglia, S., *The Complete Guide to Aromatherapy, 2nd Ed,* Perfect Potion Publisher, page 217.

[79] Johnson, S.A., *Evidence-Based Essential Oil Therapy,* Create Space Independent Publishing Platform, July 11, 2015, page 135.

[80] Lavabre, M., *Aromatherapy Workbook,* Healing Arts Press, page 84.

[81] Harris D.R., *Lavenders of Provence, The World of Aromatherapy III* - Conference proceedings, NAHA U.S.A. 1999, pages 75-81.

[82] Battaglia, S., *The Complete Guide to Aromatherapy,* Perfect Potion Publisher, page 217.

[83] Sheppard-Hanger, S., *The Aromatherapy Practitioner Reference, Manual Volume I – A-L*, Atlantic Institute of Aromatherapy 1995, page 157.

[84] Battaglia S., *The Complete Guide to Aromatherapy, 2nd Ed*, Perfect Potion Publisher, page 218.

[85] Johnson, S A., *Evidence-Based Essential Oil Therapy*, CreateSpace Independent Publishing Platform, July 11, 2015, page 133-135.

[86] Worwood, V.A., *The Fragrant Mind,* New World Library, pages 326-327.

[87] Battaglia, S., *The Complete Guide to Aromatherapy,* Perfect Potion Publisher. page 220.

[88] Schnaubelt, K., *Medical Aromatherapy: Healing With Essential Oils*, Frog Books, page 244.

[89] Schnaubelt K., *Medical Aromatherapy: Healing With Essential Oils,* Frog Books, page 244.

[90] Mailhebiau, P., *Portraits in Oils.* C.W. Daniel Publishing, page 154.

[91] Mailhebiau, P., *Portraits in Oils.* C.W. Daniel Publishing, page 158.

[92] Tisserand, R. and Young, R., *Essential Oil Safety, 2nd Ed,* Churchill Livingston Elsevier, 2014, page 329.

[93] Fischer-Rizzi, S., *Complete Aromatherapy Handbook,* Sterling Publishing Co, page 117.

[94] Battaglia, S., *The Complete Guide to Aromatherapy,* Perfect Potion Publishing, page 221.

[95] Battaglia, S., *The Complete Guide to Aromatherapy,* Perfect Potion Publishing, page 221.

[96] Tisserand, R., *International Journal of Aromatherapy, (Vol. 1, Sec.2:2)* 1988, page 2.

[97] Schnaubelt, K. , *Medical Aromatherapy: Healing With Essential Oils,* Frog Books, page 185-186.

[98] Johnson, S.A., *Evidence Based Essential Oil Therapy,* CreateSpace Independent Publishing Platform, July 11, 2015, page 142.

[99] Johnson, S.A., *Evidence-Based Essential Oil Therapy,* CreateSpace Independent Publishing Platform, July 11, 2015, Page 144.

[100] Mojay, G., *Aromatherapy for Healing the Spirit,* Healing Arts Press, page 93.

[101] Sheppard-Hanger, S., *The Aromatherapy Practitioner Reference Manual, Volume I,* Published by the Atlantic Institute of Aromatherapy 1995, page 173.

[102] Worwood, V.A. *The Fragrant Mind,* New World Library, page 328.

[103] Johnson, S.A., *Evidence-Based Essential Oil Therapy,* CreateSpace Independent Publishing Platform, July 11, 2015, page 150.

[104] Mojay G., *Aromatherapy for Healing the Spirit,* Healing Arts Press, page 92.

[105] Battaglia, S., *The Complete Guide to Aromatherapy, 2nd Ed,* Perfect Potion Publishing, page 223.

[106] Levabre, M., *Aromatherapy Workbook,* Healing Arts Press, page 81.

[107] Battaglia, S., *The Complete Guide to Aromatherapy, 3rd Ed, Vol. III,* Psyche & Subtle, Black Pepper Creative Pty LTD, page 310.

[108] Battaglia, S., *The Complete Guide to Aromatherapy 2nd Ed,* Perfect Potion Publisher, page 223.

[109] Mailhebiau, P., *Portraits in Oils,* C.W. Daniel publishing, page 194.

[110] Fischer-Rizzi, S., *Complete Aromatherapy Handbook,* Sterling Publishing Co, page 125.

[111] Zeck, R., *The Blossoming Heart: Aromatherapy for Healing and Transformation*, Aroma Tours, page 98.

[112] Fischer-Rizzi, S., *Complete Aromatherapy Handbook,* Sterling Publishing Co, page 127.

[113] Johnson, S.A., *Evidence-Based Essential Oil Therapy,* CreateSpace Independent Publishing Platform, July 11, 2015, page 150.

[114] Tisserand R. and Young R., *Essential Oil Safety, 2nd Ed.,* Churchill Livingstone, page 661-664.

[115] Schnaubelt. K., *Medical Aromatherapy*, Frog Books, page 200.

[116] Battaglia, S., *The Complete Guide to Aromatherapy,* Perfect Potion Publisher, page 283.

[117] Battaglia, S., *The Complete Guide to Aromatherapy,* Perfect Potion Publisher, page 284.

[118] Low, D., et al., *Antibacterial action of the essential oils of some Australian Myrtaceae with special references to the activity of chromatographic fractions of the oil of Eucalyptus citriodora.* Plant Medica 1974; 26: 184-189. Cited in the Aromatherapy Bates, Bob Harris, Essential oil Resource Consultants. UK 2000.

[119] Worwood, V.A., *The Fragrant Mind,* New World Library, page 307.

[120] Worwood, V.A., *The Fragrant Mind*, page 306.

[121] Battaglia, S., *The Complete Guide to Aromatherapy,* Perfect Potion Publisher, page 226.

[122] Sheppard-Hanger, S., *The Aromatherapy Practitioner Reference Manual, Volume I*, Published by the Atlantic Institute of Aromatherapy 1995, page 177.

[123] Mojay, G., *Aromatherapy for Healing the Spirit*, Healing Arts Press, page 102.

[124] Price, S. & L., *Aromatherapy for Professionals, 3rd Ed,* Churchill Livingstone, page 409.

[125] Schnaubelt, K., *Medical Aromatherapy - Healing With Essential Oils*, Frog Books, page 185.

[126] Battaglia, S., *The Complete Guide to Aromatherapy, 2nd Ed,* Perfect Potion Publisher, page 226.

[127] Worwood, V.A., *The Fragrant Mind, New World Library,* page 332-333.

[128] Battaglia, S., *The Complete Guide to Aromatherapy, 2nd Ed*, Perfect Potion Publisher, page 230.

[129] Tisseran R., Balacs, T., May Chang, *The International Journal of Aromatherapy,* 1992: 4(3), page 25-27.

[130] Battaglia, S., *The Complete Guide to Aromatherapy, 2nd Ed,* Perfect Potion Publisher, page 231.

[131] Worwood, V.A., *The Fragrant Mind,* New World Library, page 257.

[132] Battaglia, S., *The Complete Guide to Aromatherapy, 3rd Ed. Vol. III* – Psyche & Subtle, Black Pepper Creative Pty LTD, page 390.

[133] Zeck R., *The Blossoming Heart: Aromatherapy for Healing and Transformation*, Aroma Tours, page 104.

[134] Tisserand R., Young R., *Essential Oil Safety,* Churchill Livingstone. page 350.

[135] Sheppard-Hanger, S., *The Aromatherapy Practitioner Reference Manual, Volume I*, Atlantic Institute of Aromatherapy 1995, page 273.

[136] Mojay, G., *Aromatherapy for the Healing Spirit*, Healing Arts Press, page 96.

[137] Schnaubelt K., *Medical Aromatherapy: Healing With Essential Oils*, Frog Books, pages 201-202.

[138] Battaglia, S., *The Complete Guide to Aromatherapy ,2nd E.,* Perfect Potion Publisher, page 231.

[139] Battaglia, S., *The Complete Guide to Aromatherapy, 2nd Ed,* Perfect Potion Publisher, Page 232.

[140] Battaglia, S., *The Complete Guide to Aromatherapy, 2nd Ed,* Perfect Potion Publisher, page 232.

[141] Worwood, V.A., *The Fragrant Mind,* New World Library, page 338.

[142] Zeck R., *The Blossoming Heart: Aromatherapy for Healing and Transformation* , Aroma Tours, page 106.

[143] Battaglia, S., *The Complete Guide to Aromatherapy, 2nd Ed*, Perfect Potion Publisher, pages 236-237.

[144] Rischer-Rizzi S., *Complete Aromatherapy Handbook*, Sterling Publishing Co, page 142.

[145] Mojay, G., *Aromatherapy for Healing the Spirit,* Healing Arts Press, page 100.

[146] Schnaubelt, K., *Medical Aromatherapy: Healing With Essential Oils*, Frog Books, page 194.

[147] Battaglia S., *The Complete Guide to Aromatherapy 2nd Ed,* Perfect Potion Publisher, page 237.

[148] Worwood, V.A., *The Fragrant Mind,* New World Library, page 342.

[149] Zeck, R., *The Blossoming Heart: Aromatherapy for Healing and Transformation*, Aroma Tours, page 108.

[150] Sheppard-Hanger, S., *The Aromatherapy Practitioner Reference Manual, Volume 2*, Atlantic Institute of Aromatherapy 1995, page 329.

[151] Battaglia, S., *The Complete Guide to Aromatherapy, 2nd Ed,* Perfect Potion Publisher, page 321.

[152] Price S. & L., *Aromatherapy for Health Professionals, 3rd Ed*, Churchill Livingstone, page 30.

[153] Price S. & L., *Aromatherapy for Health Professionals, 3rd Ed*, Churchill Livingstone, page 448.

[154] Schnaubelt, K., *Medical Aromatherapy: Healing With Essential Oils*, Frog Books, page 92.

[155] Schnaubelt, K., *Medical Aromatherapy: Healing With Essential Oils*, Frog Books, page 194.

[156] Schnaubelt, K., *Medical Aromatherapy: Healing with Essential Oils*, Frog Books, page 203.

[157] Johnson, S.A., *Evidence Based Aromatherapy*, CreateSpace Independent Publishing Platform, July 11, 2015, page 185.

[158] Schnaubelt, K., *The Healing Intelligence of Essential Oils,* Healing Arts Press, page 82.

[159] Mojay, G., *Aromatherapy for Healing the Spirit,* Healing Arts Press, page 123.

[160] Fischer-Rizzi, S., *Complete Aromatherapy Handbook,* Sterling Publishing Co, page 208.

[161] Johnson, S.A., *Evidence Based Essential Oil Therapy,* CreateSpace Independent Publishing Platform, July 11, 2015, page 185.

[162] Battaglia, S., *The Complete Guide to Aromatherapy, 2nd Ed*, Perfect Potion Publisher, page 321.

[163] Battaglia, S., *The Complete Guide to Aromatehrapy, 2nd Ed*, Perfect Potion Publisher, page 45.

[164] Battaglia, S., *The Complete Guide to Aromatherapy, 2nd Ed*, Perfect Potion Publisher, page 249.

[165] Battaglia, S., *The Complete Guide to Aromatherapy, 2nd Ed*, Perfect Potion Publisher, page 249.

[166] Worwood, V.A., *The Fragrant Mind,* New World Library, page 351.

[167] Worwood, V.A., *The Fragrant Mind,* New World Library, page 350.

[168] Zeck, R., *The Blossoming Heart: Aromatherapy for Healing and Transformation,* Aroma Tours, page 117.

[169] Battaglia, S., *The Complete Guide To Aromatherapy, 3rd Ed., Volume III*, Psyche & Subtl, Black Pepper Creative Pty LTD, page 397.

[170] Mojay, G., *Aromatherapy for Healing the Spirit,* Healing Arts Press, page 110.

[171] Battaglia S., *The Complete Guide to Aromatherapy, 2nd Ed,* Perfect Potion Publisher, page 250.

[172] Lavabre, M., *Aromatherapy Workbook,* Healing Arts Press, page 78.

[173] Schaubelt, K., *Medical Aromatherapy: Healing With Essential Oils, Frog Books,* page 187.

[174] Worwood, V.A., *The Fragrant Mind, New World Library,* page 352.

[175] Battaglia S., *The Complete Guide To Aromatherapy, 3rd Ed, Volume III* - Psyche & Subtle, Black Pepper Creative Pty LTD, page 251.

[176] Worwood, V.A., *The Fragrant Mind,* New World Library, page 352.

[177] Mailhebiau, P., *Portraits of Oils,* C.W. Daniel Publishing, page 73.

[178] Schaubelt, K., *Medical Aromatherapy: Healing With Essential Oils, Frog Books,* page 198.

[179] Lavabre, M., *Aromatherapy Workbook,* Healing Arts Press, page 90.

[180] Tisserand, R., *Essential Oil Safety, 2nd Ed,* Churchill Livingston Elsevier, 2014, pages 412-417.

[181] Battaglia, S., *The Complete Guide To Aromatherapy, 3rd Ed, Volume 1* - Foundations & Materia Medica, Black Pepper Creative Pty LTD, pages 516-517.

[182] Mailheabiau, P., *Portraits in Oils,* C.W. Daniel publishing, page 77.

[183] Mailheabiau, P., *Portraits in Oils,* C.W. Daniel publishing, page 70.

[184] Mailheabiau, P., *Portraits in Oils,* C.W. Daniel publishing, page 80.

[185] Lavabre, M., *Aromatherapy Workbook,* Healing Arts Press, page 90.

[186] Tisserand R., Young R., *Essential Oil Safety, 2nd Ed,* Churchill Livingstone, page 414.

[187] Lavabre, M., *Aromatherapy Workbook,* Healing Arts Press, page 95.

[188] Battaglia. S., *The Complete Guide to Aromatherapy, 2nd Ed,* Perfect Potion Publisher, page 269.

[189] Mojay, G., *Aromatherapy for Healing the Spirit,* Healing Arts Press, page 120.

[190] Mojay, G., *Aromatherapy for Healing the Spirit,* Healing Arts Press. page 121.

[191] Fischer-Rizzi, S., *Complete Aromatherapy Handbook,* Sterling Publishing Co., page 212.

[192] Battaglia, S., *The Complete Guide to Aromatherapy, 2nd Ed,* Perfect Potion Publisher, page 269.

[193] Worwood, V.A., *The Fragrant Mind,* New World Library, page 261.

[194] Battaglia S., *The Complete Guide to Aromatherapy, 2nd Ed,* Perfect Potion Publisher, page 270.

[195] Sheppard-Hangar, S., *The Aromatherapy Practitioner Reference Manual, Volume II,* Published by the Atlantic Institute of Aromatherapy 1995, page 277.

[196] Battaglia, S., *The Complete Guide to Aromatherapy, 2nd Ed,* Perfect Potion Publisher, pages 271-272.

[197] Mailhebiau, P., *Portraits in Oils,* C.W. Daniel, page 119.

[198] Battaglia, S., *The Complete Guide to Aromatherapy,* Perfect Potion Publisher, page 272.

[199] Mailhebiau, P., *Portraits in Oils,* C.W. Daniel, page 123.

[200] Battaglia, S., *The Complete Guide to Aromatherapy, 2nd Ed,* Perfect Potion Publisher, page 274.

[201] Schnaubelt, K., *Medical Aromatherapy: Healing With Essential Oils,* Frog Books, page 208.

[202] Lavabre, M., *Aromatehrapy Workbook, Revised Ed,* page 81-82.

[203] Mojay, G., *Aromatherapy for Healing the Spirit, Healing Arts Press,* page 125.

[204] Worwood, V.A., *The Fragrant Mind,* New World Library, page 365-366.

[205] Fischer-Rizzi, S., *Complete Aromatherapy Handbook,* Sterling Publishing Co., page 178.

[206] Zeck, R., *The Blossoming Heart: Aromatherapy for Healing and Transformation,* Aroma Tours, page 131.

[207] Schnaubelt, K., *Medical Aromatherapy: Healing With Essential Oils,* Frog Books, page 217.

[208] Lavabre, M., *Aromatherapy Workbook,* Healing Arts Press, page 70.

[209] Battaglia S., *The Complete Guide to Aromatherapy, 2nd Ed,* Perfect Potion Publisher, page 324.

[210] Zeck, R., *The Blossoming Heart: Aromatherapy for Healing and Transformation,* Aroma Tours, page 132.

[211] Battaglia, S., *The Complete Guide to Aromatherapy, 2nd Ed,* Perfect Potion Publisher, page 324.

[212] Battaglia, S., *The Complete Guide to Aromatherapy, 2nd Ed,* Perfect Potion Publisher, page 324.

[213] Tisserand, R., & Young R., *Essential Oil Safety,* Churchill Livingstone, page 469.

[214] Battaglia, S., *The Complete Guide to Aromatherapy, 2nd Ed,* Perfect Potion Publisher, page 324.

[215] Tisserand, R., & Young R., *Essential Oil Safety,* Churchill Livingstone. page 469.

[216] Fischer-Rizzi, S., *Complete Aromatherapy Handbook,* Sterling Publishing Co, page 186.

[217] Price, L & S., *Aromatherapy for Health Professional, 2nd Ed,* Churchill Livingstone, page 20.

[218] Price, L & S., *Aromatherapy for Health Professional 2nd Ed,* Churchill Livingstone, page 394.

[219] Mojay, G., *Aromatherapy for the Healing Spirit,* Healing Arts Press, page 129.

[220] Battaglia, S., *The Complete Guide to Aromatherapy, 2nd Ed,* Perfect Potion Publisher, page 278.

[221] Battaglia, S., *The Complete Guide to Aromatherapy, 2nd Ed,* Perfect Potion Publisher, page 278.

[222] Worwood, V.A., *The Fragrant Mind,* New World Library, page 367.

[223] Zeck, R., *The Blossoming Heart: Aromatherapy for Healing and Transformation,* Aroma Tours, page 134.

Notes

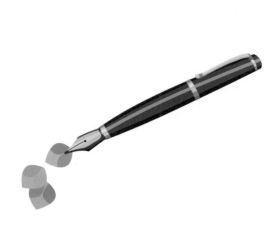

Index

A

abscess 166, 173, 179, 243, 244, 249
Absolute 26, 148, 154, 262
adrenal 43, 108, 114, 153, 214, 228, 231, 238, 250, 263, 264
Adulteration 19, 56, 169, 193
aerophagy 200
Aldehydes 19, 79, 117 119, 123, 128, 151, 161, 163, 165, 171, 183, 189, 194, 196, 198, 203, 207, 212, 258
Allergies 17, 18, 92, 146, 147, 158, 209
amenorrhea 127
analgesic 14, 80, 85, 86, 112, 117, 123, 124, 134, 135, 151, 157, 171, 178, 189, 192, 194, 218, 228, 235, 247, 257, 258
Anesthetic 121, 129, 131, 192
Angelica archangelica 103, 104
Angelica Root 43, 88, 103, 104
anorexia 108, 162, 204
Anthelmintic 117, 135, 247
Antianemic 20
Antiarthritic 165
Antibacterial 74, 84, 92, 94, 111, 117, 129, 131,135, 141, 151, 183, 207, 217, 218, 223, 233, 235, 262
antibiotic 121, 129, 192, 221
Anticatarrhal 235
anticoagulant 106, 129, 146, 148, 173, 182, 213, 221, 260
Anticonvulsive 171
Antidepressant 74, 83, 85, 112, 117, 121, 151, 153, 171, 178, 189, 192, 203, 207, 213, 218, 263

Antiemetic 123, 135
antihemorrhagic 151
Anti-inflammatory 15, 37, 39, 80, 86, 121, 145, 151, 155, 157, 178, 188, 189, 194, 203, 206, 207, 213, 218, 235, 241, 257, 258
Antimicrobial 15, 37, 123, 129, 145, 160, 171, 181, 183, 189, 218, 229, 235, 242, 247
Antineuralgic 229
Antiodontalgic 129
Antioxidant 133, 161, 187, 216, 233, 245
Antiphlogistic 145, 157, 171, 229
Antipruritic 141
Antirheumatic 140, 165, 171, 183, 194, 218, 229, 248, 257, 258
Antisclerotic 183
Antiscorbutic 183, 229
Antiseptic 86, 105, 108, 111, 112, 118, 119, 120, 123, 124, 129, 131, 135, 137, 145, 151, 161, 165, 171, 178, 179, 182, 183, 189, 191, 194, 195, 198, 203, 213, 217, 218, 223, 229, 230, 235, 240, 242, 246, 248, 250, 253, 258, 263
Antispasmodic 80, 205, 111, 112, 113, 118, 123, 129, 135, 141, 145, 151, 157, 165, 171, 183, 194, 198, 199, 207, 213, 218, 223, 235, 248, 253, 258, 263
Antisudorific 235
Antitoxic 118, 161, 171, 183, 218, 248
antitumor 181
Antitussive 145, 248, 258
antiviral 74, 84, 94, 111, 118, 124, 134, 135, 147, 171, 178, 182, 194, 207, 217, 218, 229, 233, 235, 241
Aperitif 123, 248
Aphrodisiac 106, 123, 129, 135, 137, 248, 253, 261, 263, 264

Arnica 152
Astringent 80, 129, 141, 145, 151, 161, 165, 182, 183, 189, 203, 235, 248, 258
Avocado 75

B

Bactericide 165, 171, 199, 203, 242, 248
Balsamic 139, 229, 230
Basil 42, 43, 80, 84, 90, 93, 96, 103, 110, 111, 112, 113, 115, 120
Bergamot 19, 21, 42, 73, 83, 84, 91, 93, 103, 116, 117, 119, 120, 121
Black Pepper 42, 83, 91, 93, 94, 96, 103, 122, 124, 125, 126

C

Calendula 86
Cananga odorata 103, 261, 262
Carminative 106, 111, 112, 118, 120, 123, 127, 130, 135, 157, 170, 172, 183, 189, 199, 203, 207, 213, 218, 248, 258
Carrot 105, 247
catarrh 114, 125, 173, 185, 219, 231, 237, 243
caustic 19
Cedarwood 21, 42, 43, 87, 91
cellulitis 158
Cephalic 112
chemotype 43, 103, 113, 157, 246
Cholagogue 106, 157, 172, 199, 229, 235, 248
cholera 107, 134, 137, 188
Choleretic 172, 208, 218 229, 236
cholesterol 17, 144, 214, 237, 238
cicatrizant 118, 135, 151, 157, 165, 172, 183, 213, 224, 236, 242, 248
Cinnamon 19, 21, 36, 42, 43, 71, 79, 90, 95, 127, 128, 129, 130, 132

Made in United States
Troutdale, OR
12/06/2024

25978983R00157